Anxiet
Panic At

A Guide to Overcoming Severe Anxiety, Controlling Panic Attacks and Reclaiming Your Life Again

Dr. Herman Kynaston

© Copyright 2019 - All rights reserved.

The content contained within this book may not be reproduced, duplicated or transmitted without direct written permission from the author or the publisher.

Under no circumstances will any blame or legal responsibility be held against the publisher, or author, for any damages, reparation, or monetary loss due to the information contained within this book, either directly or indirectly.

Legal Notice:

This book is copyright protected. This book is only for personal use. You cannot amend, distribute, sell, use, quote or paraphrase any part, or the content within this book, without the consent of the author or publisher.

Disclaimer Notice:

Please note the information contained within this document is for educational and entertainment purposes only. All effort has been executed to present accurate, up to date, and reliable, complete information. No warranties of any kind are declared or implied. Readers acknowledge that the author is not engaging in the rendering of legal, financial, medical or professional advice. The content within this book has been derived from various sources. Please consult a licensed professional before attempting any techniques outlined in this book.

By reading this document, the reader agrees that under no circumstances is the author responsible for any losses, direct or indirect, which are incurred as a result of the use of information contained within this document, including, but not limited to, — errors, omissions, or inaccuracies.

Table of Contents

Book Description:

Do you find yourself debilitated by anxiety that is out-of-control? Anxiety and panic can cripple your life, leaving you living in a constant state of fear. This guide puts you on a healing path.

The key to recovering from these disorders, is to first understand them. By understanding them, you begin to uncover the core reasons why your body is reacting in such severely distressing ways. Then, you can find your unique, personal formula for a full and life-changing recovery.

In *Resolving Anxiety and Panic Attacks*, I take you on an educational journey into the many facets of anxiety so that you can come to terms with your disorder. You don't have to live with the ravages of anxiety anymore. You have the power, the knowledge and the strength to recover!

In this guide you'll learn:

- Exactly what anxiety is, and why panic attacks are triggered
- The important reasons why you must focus on curing your anxiety
- Practical strategies on lowering your anxiety levels each and every day
- Physical, mental and emotional re recovery methods that work
- The damaging misconception and myths that fuel modern anxiety and panic
- How to build your personal anxiety recovery action plan

Stress doesn't have to result in unbearable anxiety and traumatic panic attacks. Learn to actively manage stress and the obstacles life throws at you – and you'll thrive.

Today is the day you reclaim your mind and your body. Discover how to stop spiraling anxiety before it negatively impacts your day. A life of calm, clarity and control is within your grasp.

Find out how to recover from anxiety and panic with this helpful guide.

Get the secrets to stress-free living now!

Introduction

Worldwide, one in six people is affected by a mental health disorder. So you are not alone in this (Ritchie & Roser, 2019). There is a difference between clinical anxiety and everyday anxiety. Everyday anxiety is normal and in often cases, it is necessary. While chronic anxiety will leave you functionally impaired. This book will not only inform you about anxiety and panic attacks but also introduce you to various methods and techniques that aid in getting rid of anxiety. It is a perfect package if you want to make long-lasting, meaningful changes in your life in a way that gets rid of anxiety. Knowledge is power, so gaining information about anxiety and panic attacks already puts you in the lead against them.

In the first chapter, we'll start with the basic knowledge of panic attacks and anxiety. The symptoms of both are pretty much the same, but there are some major differences as well. Knowing their difference and similarities can help you clearly understand your condition. Some basic ways of coping with them are also explained alongside their symptoms.

After gaining knowledge about anxiety and panic attacks in the first section, you will seek answers and ways to overcome them. The second chapter goes more in detail about the physical effects of anxiety. There are some types of anxiety which are also talked briefly about in the chapter. There are also therapies and treatments that are used to overcome and control anxiety. Their details are discussed in the chapter from where you can figure out what sort of treatment will suit you better. Some other ways of coping with anxiety are also discussed later on and they will surely prove beneficial to the reader.

The third chapter will make you aware of how interrelated physical and mental healths are. There are also details on how to improve one's physical health to influence a person's anxiety positively. You will also learn how important practicing well-being is. If you are to ignore physical health, it will cause problems for your mental health as well.

The fourth chapter will delve deep into mindfulness and its vast benefits. Mindfulness is a very powerful tool we have but don't know how to use. It can be practiced through meditation techniques, etc. It makes us see things more clearly than ever before. Practicing Mindfulness will arm you against any anxiety and panic attacks. In this chapter, it is explained in detail what it means and what are its advantages.

In the fifth chapter, we will learn about meditation and how can it help manage anxiety. We first start off by knowing what it is. You also have got to know its benefits and various techniques from which one can pick according to their choice. We will also learn the accurate posture you should have during meditation. We will learn how mediation reinforces our brain to stave off anxiety and panic attacks. It is a long road but a successful one for sure. Besides helping us out with anxiety and panic disorder, meditation has numerous other benefits for our body and mind.

The sixth chapter will explore the meaning behind self-love and its importance in fighting anxiety. Our battle with anxiety has to start from a positive ground. We first have to be fully comfortable and respectful towards ourselves. You will also find out how lack of self-love can actually breed anxiety.

Opening about anxiety is not an easy task but could be very helpful against anxiety. How to go about the whole process is talked about in detail in the seventh chapter. You will also learn how to evaluate your therapist and choose the right one. In this chapter, there are also guidelines for people who have just recently become aware of their anxiety and now they want to seek help. It will give them knowledge about things to consider when talking to someone about mental health, what you should accept and be prepared for. There is also information about talk therapy there.

In the eighth chapter, we address the misunderstanding about anxiety. Despite affecting so many people, it remains a different experience for all of them. There are also common mistakes pointed out in that chapter which we'll go into detail the mistakes that make our anxiety worse.

The ninth chapter is about where we talk about putting our foot down and start to incorporate practices into our life which will help you get rid of anxiety and panic attacks. We will learn how to manage our responses. It is basically a comprehensive listing of all the things you should be avoiding or adapting to lead a healthy lifestyle free of anxiety.

Chapter 1: What is anxiety?

"The rest of your life will not be mastered in just one day

Relax and master the day

Then keep doing that every single day."

What to know about Anxiety?

Anxiety is caused by any stress you are going through. It is a feeling of dread which overcomes you about a future event. Nearly 30% of adults experience anxiety at some point in their lives. Anxiety disorders are treatable. With the right treatment, it could lead to a productive and healthy lifestyle by overcoming your anxiety.

Anxiety has a number of symptoms which are: irrational worry, distress, and fear. Anxiety can also overcome a person gradually. It usually occurs in anticipation of a stressful situation. Anxiety disorder is when you experience these feelings on an extreme level and they interfere with your daily life. This jittery feeling on a small scale is normal for everybody, but if they last typically more than six months or so, then they could be due to a disorder.

You experience irrational fear all the time and what motivated you to do something better or be prepared more has turned into a huge distraction. Anxiety, if left untreated could take a turn for the worse. It starts off with you being unmotivated and then outright stop doing things you once enjoyed. Then it leads to an inability to do normal tasks without a feeling of fear.

Anxiety can affect a person at any age. It is more common in women than men, according to the American psychiatric association.

Anxiety is a natural response of the body since the early days where man was all about survival. The onset of triggers for dangers allowed us to undertake necessary action on whether to fight or hide. Anxiety sets off many alarms in our body where we can physically feel the tension of the prevailing situation. Sweating and racing-heartbeat are common symptoms that allow being better in tune with the surrounding. This feeling of danger releases adrenaline which is a chemical of the brain that triggers acute stress response of our body. This response is also called the fight or flight response. It is a psychological reaction that occurs due to a perceived threat to survival or dangerous situation.

For us humans now, things have developed manifold. We are not running for our lives. We don't need a trigger of our fight or flight response while going about our daily activities. The nervous or anxious feeling before something important is a testament to our ancient survival tactic.

Anxiety has several levels. It could be mild, moderate, or severe, mostly ranging from jittery feeling to extreme fear. Panic attacks are always on a serious level where you are not able to focus on anything else. Your body will basically be on fight or flight mode. It is one of the most common forms of emotional disorder.

How you experience anxiety could be totally different from the other person. Some people have nightmares while others have to sit through a barrage of painful memories or thoughts. All in all, it is very exhausting in whatever shape or form anxiety affects a person. Some of the general symptoms are:

- Rapid breaths
- Nausea
- A headache or trouble in focusing
- Insomnia
- Increase in heart rate

This funny feeling called anxiety could be a lifesaver if it comes and goes at the right time. If it decides to stay, then it could be very harmful to the mental health of a person.

Unfortunately, the causes of anxiety are unknown as of yet. A lot of factors directly contribute to it though. Development of a person from their childhood is a huge factor. There could be a mishandled event which led to the development of anxiety. Psychological, environmental, and genetics are also some factors. Anxiety disorders can run in the family also.

What to know about Panic Attacks?

A panic attack is an unexpected and intense feeling of overwhelming fear. They entail various physical symptoms as well such as racing heartbeat, nausea, and the shortage of breath. A panic attack is a frightening experience both mentally and physically. Physically, panic attacks can cause your knees to go weak and have chest pain. It can also cause dizziness, and for a second you may think you are having a heart attack. It only lasts for a while, but it can leave you really terrified and wary that another one might be coming in the future.

When this situation keeps on happening frequently, then it is classified as a panic disorder. A panic disorder can cause a person to avoid a certain situation for the fear of panic attacks. They will eventually realize it is not the situation they were avoiding but the panic attack itself.

Lately, panic attacks have been categorized into expected and unexpected types by (DSM-5) Diagnostic and Statistical Manual of Mental Disorders. ("DSM-5 Criteria for Diagnosing Panic Disorder", 2019)[1].

- Expected panic attacks are usually caused by external stress factors, such as phobias.
- Unexpected ones don't have an obvious identifiable cause.

Panic and anxiety attack may seem similar because they share a lot of emotional and physical symptoms. It is difficult to differentiate between them sometimes.

You can also experience both at the same time. An example of it is, if you are experiencing anxiety about a stressful event, it will wind up into panic attacks

[1] DSM-5 Criteria for Diagnosing Panic Disorder. (2019). Retrieved from https://www.verywellmind.com/diagnosing-panic-disorder-2583930

on the arrival of the said event. Main differences are that panic attacks are mostly out of the blue. Anxiety could be due to an upcoming situation that you deem stressful or threatening.

A panic attack is different from an anxiety attack. Here are some symptoms of an anxiety attack:

- Dizziness
- Dry mouth
- Sweating
- Chills or hot flashes
- Worry and fear
- Restlessness
- Numbness

If you learn to manage your anxiety, then you can further go on to completely avoid a panic attack. There are many techniques to calm your mind and body whenever you notice that a panic attack may be arising. The oncoming symptoms will eventually fade away and you would have successfully avoided a panic attack.

Coping with a panic attack

Coping with the feeling of panic is the first step to manage panic attack successfully.

Some anxiety managing techniques are here below; they will not only help in warding off the panic attack but also successfully take control of the anxious feeling.

Focus on Breathing

The first step to take is to focus on and regulate your breathing. Irregular breathing can make your symptoms even worse. Take a count of slow and deep breaths to help calm yourself.

Stop your train of thoughts

Whatever is going on your mind, try and put a halt on them. Throw them out of the metaphorical window. Only focus on yourself and put yourself in control of your own thoughts.

Positive thoughts

Assign your mind a happy place to wander into whenever you are in the situation. It will help you eventually realize that nothing is as bad as it seems right now.

Put yourself first

Don't feel bad about asking for help or leaving the situation. If you deem it necessary at that time to help you, then don't second guess yourself.

Practice these strategies if you have symptoms of anxiety. You won't get efficient with dealing right away as it is a gradual process.

Confronting your fear is very important. Don't let fear of a panic attack control you. Ride out the attack because, in the end, you will know that nothing life threatening happened. It can help you understand the situation better.

Having someone close will also help; someone that can steadily assure you throughout it. These situations once experienced will help mentally prepare you better for these episodes until you finally learn to overcome it.

Stress, Depression, and Anxiety

Anxiety and depression are related to each other. If you have the former disorder, you will be likely to have depression as well. They can occur separately too.

If a person ignores anxiety and depression throughout their life, it will likely result in a physical health issue. Mostly heart-related problems arise due to untreated anxiety or depression.

What happens to the brain during anxiety?

Let's take the help of science to understand anxiety better. Brain chemistry also plays a vital role. Researchers believe that as a result of anxiety, the area of the brain in charge of fear may be affected. So here are parts of the brain affected by anxiety. (I. Martin, J. Ressler, Binder & B. Nemeroff, 2013)[2]

Amygdala (It stores memories of emotional experiences and frightening events that occurred in our life.) People with anxiety have extremely sensitive amygdala. It will also react to non-threatening situations for them.

Hippocampus (It has the main role in processing emotions. It also deals with long term memories.) Hippocampus is also smaller in depressed people.

Locus Ceruleus (It determines which brain stimuli are worthy of attention.)

The prefrontal cortex (It is the part of the brain involved in making decisions, passing judgments, and problem-solving.) It can turn down fear response and is responsible for storing memories of situations of overcoming any fear. These two factors are key to treatment of anxiety.

Ways to reduce stress

- Listening to music will help greatly in dealing with a stressful situation. It has the power to calm down your brain, so it is fresh and ready for tasks ahead. Listen to calming music in a stressful situation could lead to being more productive than before.
- Give yourself a pep talk. Be your own boss. Sometimes, your only option is to rely on yourself. Stand in front of the mirror and try talking

[2] I. Martin, E., J. Ressler, K., Binder, E., & B. Nemeroff, C. (2013). The Neurobiology of Anxiety Disorders: Brain Imaging, Genetics, and Psychoneuroendocrinology. Retrieved from https://www.ncbi.nlm.nih.gov/pmc/articles/PMC3684250/

to yourself. It may seem crazy to others, but it is a very good technique to improve your thinking and get a clear head. Don't worry about seeming crazy; you have to build a little resilience and care less about what others think. It can go a long way in building confidence and fighting off stress caused by behaviors and the opinions of others.

- Some people, when under stress, tend to stop eating while others eat a lot. Both extreme behaviors are very damaging to health and only tend to make our stress levels worse than before.
- When under stress, all you need is a bit of perspective. You must ring up the person who can put things into perspective for you and give you a gentle slap of reality. Sometimes that's all it takes for stress to subside.
- Laughter is truly the best medicine. Laughing off a stressful situation is often enough for us to get out of whatever had us down. Laughter releases endorphins that will lighten one's mood. Try to incorporate laughter into your daily life.
- Green tea has been advised to be taken when in a stressful situation. It truly has a calming effect, not to mention the healthy dose of antioxidants.
- Lack of sleep is a straight one-way ticket to stress. Regular lack of sleep has an alarming number of bad effects on your mind and body. So always make sure to get the recommended good eight hours or so of sleep in the most comfortable environment that you can make for yourself. Yes, naps are revolutionary but have you laid down in bed under the covers and had a good night of sleep? It is the most effective stress buster out there.
- Short breaths are a cause of stress while deep breaths will oxygenate your whole body. It will sharpen your focus as it clears your mind.

What you call an anxiety attack may build up slowly. It is the hugely crushing feeling of worry and fear. The feeling of distress only gets worse as the event that troubles you gets nearer.

Anxiety can lead to addictive behavior. For example, alcohol is a sedative, it helps slows the activity of the brain and in turn, we feel relaxed and calm. What it is, is not a solution to get out of feeling anxious. However, most people suffering from anxiety in a social situation tend to abuse alcohol to help them calm down and relax. If this goes on regularly, it can lead to alcohol addiction. Alcohol will end up doing more harm than good because chronic addiction to it must be treated first.

Anxiety is directly related to avoidance behavior. It could lead you to separate yourself from important tasks out of fear. You will tend to avoid situations that worsen anxiety symptoms and are a cause of triggering them. These situations could be your school, workplace, or even the company of some people. It can prove to be detrimental, not for you but also the people surrounding you.

As they say, "adventure is dangerous, but a routine is lethal." For someone living a monotonous life in the same routine, falling into depression is pretty easy. You have to shake things up and try not to stick to routine too much. Take a break from work. Go on vacation and spend quality time with your loved ones. Don't let your work rule you. Take it from wise old people. They always advise the young to make memories and not run after money. I think it is high time that we finally listen to them.

Chapter 2: Effects of Anxiety and How to Deal with it

"Thinking about the future is not the cause of anxiety. It is the want to control it."

Treatments and Therapies

Therapies for an anxiety disorder:

Cognitive behavior therapy:

One of the best ways to treat anxiety. Anxiety and panic attacks are a result of thinking about the future and what could be the disastrous implications of it. People are made aware that their thinking is what causes the physical symptoms in the first place, so it is better to stop right then and there. (C. Butler, E. Chapman & M.Forman, 2006)[3]

Exposure therapy:

As the name suggests, this therapy will make you confront the situation that you run away from due to their stress and anxiety-inducing effects. The idea is that through repeated, continued exposure, you can overcome the feeling of dread that settles upon you when facing those kinds of situations. Your sense of control over the particular situation will gradually increase.

---

[3] C. Butler, A., E. Chapman, J., & M.Forman, E. (2006). The empirical status of cognitive-behavioral therapy: A review of meta-analyses [Ebook]. Science Direct.

There are also medications available for the treatment of anxiety and panic attacks.

Treatment for anxiety:

There is not one single test that is undertaken to prove that you could have anxiety. It is done through a long process of mental health evaluations, questionnaires, and physical exams. There are also tests and scales that will find out the level of anxiety a person has. To start off, on your first session, you will undergo a psychological evaluation. You will be asked about your feeling and thoughts.

Experiencing more than one condition at once is possible. Untreated anxiety will worsen over time. If left like that, to worsen, it will be more difficult to treat. It is difficult to distinguish between an anxiety disorder or a really bad day. However, these are some of the signs that you should absolutely not ignore and head out to seek help.

- Your constant worry is affecting your everyday routine life. You feel as though you would be able to perform them more efficiently if not for the nagging thoughts of your brain.
- You have started relying on unhealthy coping mechanisms to escape from your own thoughts and fears.
- Once little worries and nagging thoughts have grown to genuinely distress you now to the point of having suicidal thoughts.

Once you have decided that it's time to seek help, then first comes the visit to a physician. It is to make sure that anxiety is not due to a physical condition. Once it's proved to not be a physical case, then you will be referred to mental health specialists.

A psychologist is a mental health professional who will use counseling only to treat mental health conditions. A psychiatrist is a licensed doctor who will treat mental health conditions through medications and other treatments. They are both able to diagnose a person.

Finding the right mental health care provider is very important. You should be able to feel comfortable in their presence enough to open up about yourself. If that is not the case, then there is no point in seeking therapy. If you are determined to go to proper therapy, then seek the right kind of help from the right person.

Treatment of anxiety yields its result gradually and you need to be patient to see them. Following the direction of your healthcare provider is the key to finding a long term cure for anxiety. Be sure to take your medications regularly and don't skip appointments. Following through both of these tasks will help keep your anxiety disorder symptoms at bay.

Treatment for anxiety is a 24/7 type of task. While treatments, medications, and counseling will yield positive results in due time, there are some simple lifestyle changes that you could acquire which will help in fighting off anxiety.

You must make efforts to know what triggers your anxiety. So consciously you can work around those symptoms and try to come up with a solution preferably better than avoiding it altogether. Your mental health care provider will help you with specific coping strategies against those triggers. So, next time you are prepared to deal with your anxiety.

Writing down your behaviors about certain experiences and situations will ultimately help your mental healthcare provider gain more insight into your condition. He will then make a more effective treatment plan for you based on that knowledge.

It is recommended to find a support group near you. Listening to them and talking with them throws a positive outlook on the whole scenario. It means you are not alone, That more people are facing the same issues. You will be more determined than before to continue your struggle against your anxiety.

Some people experiencing anxiety tend to shy away from friends and family. You must know that it will only make your anxiety way worse than before. Relying on people is an important step to take for people suffering from a mental disorder. You have to know that people are there to support you and

they are not going to go anywhere. Distancing yourself from ones you love could lead to a more anxious feeling such as you constantly wondering what they are going to think of you. You will only end up making assumptions in your head that are far away from reality and they will end up hurting you more.

Effects and Types of Anxiety

Some of the effects that anxiety could have on our body besides the physical symptoms that manifest are:

- The cardiovascular system is seriously affected by constant worry and anxiety. Increased heartbeat and palpitations along with chest pains only spell trouble for you in the long run.
- Anxiety can also directly affect the digestive system. It can cause diarrhea or vomiting in case of extreme anxiety.
- If you frequently suffer from anxiety, then it can take a toll on your immune system as well. Adrenaline is released in your body whenever you experience a severe case of anxiety. It can boost your immune system for a little while, but over time, it will have bad effects on your immune system.
- Muscle fatigue and tension in the body are caused by experiencing anxiety and panic attacks.

Types of anxiety disorder:

Generalized Anxiety Disorder (GAD):

- Generalized anxiety disorder is when even mundane daily activities can induce feelings of anxiety in a person. The situation doesn't call for that much stress as a person experiencing this disorder may feel. Stress and constant worry will cause adverse effects on a person's health. They may experience insomnia and upset stomach.

Obsessive Compulsive Disorder (OCD):

- It is a mental disorder where there is a constant barrage of unwanted, intrusive thoughts. They will cause one to develop obsessive behaviors where they will do a certain thing over and over again. These compulsive behaviors will only provide a short term relief, but the person with the disorder will be doing them to get rid of intrusive thoughts in the first place.
- Without performing these routines will result in a great deal of distress for the person, so they carry on with this behavior.

Agoraphobia:

- People suffering from this disorder presume certain situations or places to be the cause of their stress. They experience mortification just by the thought of them. So, they try to avoid them as much as possible as it can lead to them having a panic attack.

Post-traumatic stress disorder (PTSD):

- PTSD is usually caused after a very nightmarish situation.
- Some disturbing experiences such as war, an assault, or an accident are some of the main causes of post-traumatic stress disorder. After a large scale natural disaster hits, one of the most mental disorder cases to arise is PTSD. Some of its symptoms are insomnia, nightmares, and flashbacks of troubled times.

Separation Anxiety Disorder:

- It mainly occurs in younger children. This type of anxiety prevails when a child is separated from their parents. Most outgrow this anxiety around 18 months. It is a normal childhood condition. In some of the cases, children continue to depict versions of it that might become an issue as it causes a disturbance in their daily routine. For example, children refusing to perform well in school in the early years just because of this disorder.

Selective mutism:

- Some children refuse to engage themselves when placed in specific situations or places. They outright don't talk. This disorder is called selective mutism and it can have a huge effect on daily routine and the person himself if not recognized and left untreated. An example is that they will not say a word at school but talk just fine at home.

Panic disorder:

- Panic disorder is a frequent occurrence of panic attacks. They could be sudden or a result of a gradual buildup of anxiety.

Phobias:

- Phobia is when a certain object, a specific situation or place can trigger severe anxiety in a person when they encounter it. They have a mighty need to avoid it at all costs. Some examples are claustrophobia (fear of being in cramped or small spaces) or coulrophobia (fear of clowns).

How to cope with anxiety

Nutrition and Anxiety

One might wonder whether what we eat can help us with our anxiety. Well, the answer is simple, yes. Depression and anxiety go hand in hand. If you set out to cure one of them, it will indirectly cure the other one as well.

Complex carbohydrates are metabolized relatively slowly. So, it means that blood sugar levels will not be spiking and it will help keep the body relax.

Skipping meals is a big no-no. When you are dealing with anxiety disorder especially, it all becomes a game of blood sugar level. Fluctuating blood sugar levels are directly related to mood swings.

The standard American diet cannot directly cause anxiety, but it can definitely make it worse. As it is full of sugar and fat, it is not very good for your physical health as well. A random sugar high and crash will cause shaking and tension in the body. It will severely impair a body's ability to deal with stress.

Anxiety relieving diet

- Try food rich in magnesium. They include Spanish, legumes, nuts, and seeds.
- Oysters, liver, beef and egg yolks should be included in the diet as they are rich in zinc. They are proven to be helpful in reducing anxiety.
- Omega-3s help improve depression and anxiety both. Their main source is salmon.
- Avocados and almonds are foods enriched in vitamin B.
- Those 'feel good' foods that release neurotransmitters such as dopamine and serotonin are safe.
- Try to take foods enriched in antioxidants. A lowered antioxidant state is thought to be correlated to anxiety. Some foods enriched in antioxidants are beans, pecans, fruits, and berries. Especially turmeric and ginger have both antioxidant and anti-anxiety properties.

Random spikes in blood sugar levels will cause moody behavior and depression. Try to eat regularly, so you avoid feeling negative altogether. Neglecting your personal needs could not only physically drain you but could be exponentially bad for your mental health especially if you suffer from anxiety disorder.

Natural remedies for anxiety:

Exercise, meditation, and yoga are excellent techniques and they are discussed further in detail in upcoming chapters.

Some other natural remedies are:

Acupuncture is the ancient Chinese medical practice of inserting very thin needles at certain points of the body. It is believed to be effective in fighting off anxiety.

Kava is a herb that comes from a crushed root of a Polynesian shrub. Some studies have proved that it helps in the treatment of anxiety although there is not definite proof. It is still a natural thing and has no adverse side effects when taken into moderation.

Lavender is believed to have a calming and soothing scent. It is used for aromatherapy. It can help soothe frayed nerves, but it doesn't actually treat the disorder itself.

Breathing exercise: it is better to keep your eyes closed. Shutting down your vision could relieve your brain from so much activity and it will also help in tune your other senses.

- First of all, inhale through the nose slowly and gently. Try to take as much a deep breath as you can.
- Exhale through the mouth just as you inhaled, slowly and deeply.

It is also a good technique to count to a number. It just helps focus on your breathing more.

"Nothing can bring you peace but yourself."

Ralph Waldo Emerson

Dealing with Anxiety Everyday

Doing breathing exercises will help you become more confident in your ability to fend off panic attacks.

Exercise and a well-balanced diet could do wonders to improve mood. Once your lifestyle is positive, then your thoughts start to become positive as well. You have to make that choice though.

Caffeine alcohol and smoking make the panic and anxiety disorders worse so try to stay away from those as much as possible. Make better health choices. (Connolly, 2018)[4]

Yoga, meditation are some of the relaxation and stress management techniques that will put your mind at peace. They are ultimately related to positive attitude and will greatly prove beneficial to people experiencing an anxiety disorder.

Getting a good night sleep and eating at appropriate times are the simplest things that you can easily embed into your life. They will yield incredibly positive results in your life and make it much more productive and smoother.

Living and coping with anxiety is no piece of cake. It drains your energy that you would much rather put in something productive. However, it is no use to hide from anxiety. You must accept it at one stage and learn to deal with it. If you remain determined and preserved, then you can eventually overcome it as well. There are some simple steps you can take to better deal with anxiety.

Try to collect as much information as you can about your condition. Don't hesitate to ask your doctor as well. Don't shy away from making healthy choices for your life. Some people may call them old style as compared to this haphazard lifestyle which is very common now. Today's lifestyle of being blinded by the success of money and fame could lead to detrimental effects on one's mental wellbeing.

---

[4] Connolly, M. (2018). Anxiety and Caffeine - this stimulant in coffee or tea may fuel anxiety. Retrieved from https://www.psycom.net/anxiety-and-caffeine

Chapter 3: Physical Health and Anxiety

"It all begins with you. If you do not care for your own self, you will not be strong enough to take care of anything in life" - Leon Brown

Relation of Physical and Mental health

Mind and body should not be thought of as separate from one another. They are both responsible for the proper functioning of a human being. If one health is declining, then there is definitely going to be an effect on the other.

People suffering from distress are 32% more likely to die from cancer than those who don't have self-induced distress about the disease. ("Physical health and mental health", 2019)[5]. Schizophrenia is also a mental disorder that doubles the risk of heart disease and increases the risk of respiratory disease by three times. Depression has been associated directly to heart problems.

This chapter would help in the realization that physical health should also be taken care of if you suffer from mental health issues.

Anxiety Disorders

There is not one identifiable cause of anxiety which will pinpoint its exact origin. However, there are some factors that are identified by researchers of mental health. According to them, these circumstances make us prone to anxiety disorders.

---

[5] Physical health and mental health. (2019). Retrieved from https://www.mentalhealth.org.uk/a-to-z/p/physical-health-and-mental-health

Anxiety disorders are more often than not appear to run in families. Although, there is no proof that genetic factors are involved. It may just be that environmental factors surrounding that particular household that are the cause.

Personality is the major factor in determining how we perceive everyday life and our behavior to our environment. More often, introverts are prone to anxiety than extroverts. Some people are perfectionists and some like to just get things done. Generally, low self-esteem arises from overthinking and poor coping mechanisms. All these things are mostly found in people who suffer from depression.

Neurotransmitters' lack or excess is also directly related to anxiety. Imbalance in them causes the anxiety-producing pathways to react more than normal.

Some illnesses such as long term heart disease or diabetes are sometimes the cause of an anxiety disorder. It might not be illness itself but a person's reaction to it. A feeling of helplessness can quickly bring on depression. If this is not identified and dealt with, then it will soon develop into anxiety.

Some hormonal gland problems have been directly linked to causing stress and anxiety.

Caffeine can make anxiety symptoms worse. Alcohols and drugs are also known to enhance the anxiety of the user.

Sometimes, a single event can turn it upside down for you. The occurrence of a horrible event may have had caused huge distress upon a person. Its consequences could be detrimental to a person's mental health. For example, abuse, the death of a loved one, a relationship cut-off, hectic jobs, etc. are some common events that have a huge impact on a person. It could also lead to developing severe anxiety.

Lifestyle Factors Affecting Both Types of Health

Here are some of the things you can do that would help in improving both your mental and physical health.

Diet

Ever heard the phrase "you are what you eat." It is true even though we eat every day, it's a common activity and we don't really pay attention to it, except those who are health freaks. It is a good thing to be concerned about what you are eating. Eating is one of the most important things needed for survival after all.

A good healthy diet will keep us healthy and the opposite will bring on a number of problems that make themselves appear over time. A healthy diet of fats, proteins, vitamins, minerals, and carbohydrates is essential to nutrition. The diet we intake can influence our physical health and it becomes pretty apparent to us over time. What we eat can directly influence mental health disorders such as Alzheimer's and depression.

Exercise

Any kind of positive physical activity is very important for our physical health. What we don't pay attention to is how it is necessary for our mental health as well. It is proven by research that doing exercise will release endorphins in the brain. They are feel-good chemicals that lift the mod. They will increase your awareness and energy. Even just walking for a while has an amazing impact on one's mood.

By physical activity, it means expending energy by movements that involve your muscles. Even just doing normal chores around the house will improve your mental health and you will have a clean house in the end. Exercise is a win-win situation for your body and brain.

Smoking

It is pretty much established that smoking is extremely harmful to your health. The funny thing is most people claim to do it for mental health reasons. They feel like they can effectively reduce their depression and stress through it. But it is only a short term solution and in the long run, its consequences outweigh whatever momentary benefits it presents.

People with depression are more likely to smoke than other people.

Cigarettes contain nicotine. It is a chemical that disrupts and alters chemicals in our brain. People with depression have lower levels of dopamine. Dopamine is responsible for inducing the positive feeling in our brains. Nicotine temporarily increases the production of dopamine. In the long run, it severely affects the natural ability to produce more dopamine in the future. So a person winds up addicted to smoking just because they think it is the answer to their troubles.

Effects of Anxiety on Physical Health

Anxiety has a considerable effect on our physical health not only for short term but also in the long run. If it, unfortunately, goes on for long, a person could develop chronic physical conditions.

When a person starts to get anxious or stressed, the brain sends signals to the body. Our body ends up releasing adrenaline and cortisol. Both of these are stress hormones. They are only good for the body when we are in actual danger, not for everyday life situations.

Some of the negative effects anxiety can have on our body systems involve:

1. **Respiratory systems**

Hyperventilation is when a person has difficulty breathing. It becomes shallow and rapid. This occurs during anxiety. During this whole process, the body intakes much more oxygen to supply to the brain. They often began gasping for breath as they feel a heightened need for it. Some of its accompanying symptoms are weakness, dizziness, lightheadedness, and the feeling that you are about to faint.

1. **Cardiovascular system**

As anxiety can change the breathing pattern so directly, it will also affect the heartbeat too. It can cause a change in heart rate and circulation.

This all is to cater for the fight-or-flight response your brain has told your body to do. Your muscles will start getting more oxygen and nutrients because it makes your body think you are in a fight with someone when really you will only be stressed for a test.

Hot flashes can also occur in the body. It happens when our blood vessels narrow, which is called vasoconstriction. Vasoconstriction affects the temperature of the body. After then, the body starts sweating apparently to cool down but then you end up feeling cold.

2. Immune system

All the boost our body gets from anxiety is short-lived and for the long run, it messes up our immune system badly.

People with more serious anxiety disorders tend to get more flu and colds.

3. Digestive system

Cortisol is a stress hormone. It is released during any situation where we are threatened or when under distress. Its function is to block off the processes of the body that are nonessential in a fight-or-flight situation. As digestion is not particularly needed in a threatening situation, it turns that down as well. Adrenaline is the culprit too as it blocks the blood flow and stomach muscles relax. As a result, you feel nausea and lose your appetite. It also causes diarrhea and you feel like your stomach is upset. There is also some research to suggest that depression can cause irritable bowel syndrome.

4. Urinary

So during a fight-or-flight response, it is natural to have an empty bladder. So that it would make us run faster. That is why we tend to get an increased urge to urinate whenever we are anxious or under stress.

Simple Practices for Wellbeing

One of the best things that you can do to practice wellbeing is exercise. Putting your body under stress will reduce the stress off your brain.

You don't have to exercise like everybody else. Any other physical activity will be just as good if not better. You will enjoy it also so overall it will become an activity that you will look forward to and enjoy doing.

There are supplements proven to reduce anxiety and depression. Some of them are

- Lemon balm
- Omega-3 fatty acids
- Ashwagandha
- Green tea
- Valerian
- Kava Kava

Candles are great for aesthetic and lighting up your mood. The scented ones or essential oils will help reduce the feeling of stress and help produce a peaceful effect on your surroundings.

Aromatherapy is the use of scents to make your mood better. Some of the soothing scents are

- Rose
- Sandalwood
- Lavender

High dosage of caffeine can promote anxiety. Especially if you notice signs that after caffeine intake, you get jittery, then consider cutting it out of your life. It can be healthy in moderate amounts. You should test out your threshold for caffeine intake and notice if you experience anxiety more afterward.

Talking about your feelings isn't always easy. Finding an outlet for your feelings and thoughts is a very healthy way to deal with them. One of those outlets is writing. Writing about your feelings and thoughts can help you positively confront them as well as letting them out. Bottling up your feelings is never a healthy thing.

Writing about both negative and positive things in your life is a progressive habit and it will help you grow as a person. By recording negative thoughts, you are facing them in a clearer perspective. By writing positive things, you are being thankful for their existence.

Chewing gum. Believe it or not, it has a number of physical and mental health benefits. People who chewed gum has a greater sense of wellbeing according to a study. They experience lower levels of stress. Chewing gum makes more blood flow to the brain. It produces brain waves that are the same as of those people who are relaxed (Smith, Chaplin & Wadsworth, 2012)[6]. Did you ever observe that whenever something stressful is going on a person tends to chew gum more aggressively? Well, a recent study found that stress relief happens more when gum is chewed more aggressively.

Don't underestimate the power of friendship. Having a good friend is a treasure. Spending time around your loved ones, who are there to support you will give a feeling of belonging. It will help reduce depression. People with few friends are also more likely to suffer from anxiety. Spend time on your relationships. Try connecting with people; however, you are comfortable.

Laughter is good for your health. It relieves stress and tension in your body.

Listen to your favorite tunes.

Having a pet can give you a sense of purpose and keep you active. It will also be a great company. These are all the best ways to combat anxiety.

---

[6] Smith, A., Chaplin, K., & Wadsworth, E. (2012). Chewing gum, occupational stress, work performance and wellbeing.

Learn to stay on top of your schedule. Having things burden up on you will likely cause a lot of stress. Simply don't put off what can be done today for tomorrow.

Keep yourself productively busy, try not to limit yourself by thinking that you are not up to doing certain hobbies. Learn to approach life with an open mind. Having a number of interests and pursuing those staves off anxiety.

If you are in a position to give back to the world, then do so. Simple volunteer work is great if you can do so. Even a smile or thank you counts a lot in the rash world today.

The best thing you can do for your mind is not to overthink. Learn to be in the moment and be mindful as explained in the previous chapter.

Chapter 4: The Wonders of Mindfulness

"By living deeply in the present moment, we can understand the past better and we can prepare for a better future." - Thich Nhat Hanh

Nothing changes for you if you don't take the first step. Making up your mind to stand up to whatever is holding you back is when you will truly make progress. If you are on medications for anxiety and doing every other thing there is to get better; it won't make a real difference until you practice self-care yourself.

Anxiety disorder is not as simple as a single feeling of being on edge. It is a culmination of different factors that make a person behaves the way they do.

What is Mindfulness?

Like the word itself, it means the mind is only occupied to what is happening in the present. The mind's main focus is on what is happening in the space you are occupying and the present task at hand. This seems like a minor thing to have such a fuss about but it is actually really important. There are so many people other than those with anxiety who can't seem to focus or concentrate on the present. Usually, the mind veers to the future or the past. This is the root cause of anxiety and panic attacks.

Mindfulness can make us snap to reality no matter where our mind diverges to. Mindfulness is an innate ability that some have mastered more than others. It is not a new skill or discovery. It makes people better equipped to pay attention and enable them to stay more focused than others. You can also learn to hone this natural ability. It can prove to be significant for anyone. Using mindfulness to beat the panic is one of the most effective methods. Some of the methods to improve your mindfulness are through different techniques of meditation. Some of which are:

- Lying down
- Walking
- Being seated

Mindfulness is different for everyone. It doesn't mean that a bunch of people who practice it more consciously become more alike in personality. Mindfulness can make you become more of who you already are.

Mindfulness is guaranteed to improve your relationships, and have a positive impact on work and health. Life can be more meaningful without the unnecessary stress, won't it? You will be able to see things more clearly and respond better. Simply put, it will make your lifestyle more efficient. You will be able to approach your daily experiences with open-mindedness and be gentler toward yourself too.

Benefits of Mindfulness

1. Some of the benefits of mindfulness:
2. Improve sleep quality. You will see results just after a little while of practicing; it will boost your body's immune system.
3. It will directly reduce anxiety and stress. It is a sure way to increase positive emotions that will help you prevent relapsing from stress.
4. It can increase gray matter in some of our brain areas that are: empathy, memory, learning, and emotional regulation. So, that means you can get better in all of those things by just practicing mindfulness. ("A Little Meditation Goes a Long Way", 2019)
5. Mindfulness will let us stop worrying about unnecessary things, so we get a chance to see the real picture. It can lead to one being more altruistic and compassionate not only to others but to themselves also.

6. One of the things anxiety chips away from us is our self-esteem and confidence. Mindfulness can help you regain that and build a much more positive image of yourself. You are then more likely to act on your values.
7. It can also help in dealing with past trauma. Since mindfulness means to survive in the now, you will become more resilient about your past. It can help with anxiety disorders that stem from past experiences.
8. Mindfulness can help you in every walk of life. It can help you with decision making and increasing creativity. These two things combined spell progress in your workplace.
9. It will reduce stress for parents so they would pay better attention to their kids. In schools, it has very effective and positive results for students. Teaching kids mindfulness can help them with behavior problems and aggression.

Mindfulness practices:

Meditation is a practice that has numerous mental health benefits despite seemingly being a simple thing. We gain more awareness and insight through it. It can notably help to reduce stress and increase productiveness. Mindfulness will suspend the judgment element of your brain and you get to focus on other things.

Mindfulness has a number of factors:

- Pay attention to your senses at the moment. Otherwise, you would miss their signals and easily let your mind wander.
- In case of experiencing an overwhelming panic attack, pay attention to your breathing.
- Throughout the day, reserve some moments for practicing mindfulness. It will help you clear your head and focus more.

- Drilling positive thought patterns into your brain consists of recognizing that our thoughts and emotions are not bigger than us. They do not define us.

Here are several exercises that will help you acquire the necessary mindfulness skills.

Body Scan

In this exercise, you are expected to feel each and every part of the body separately.

Raisin Exercise

You are to utilize each of your senses, one by one, to pay attention to a raisin. For example, the feel of it by your hands or its smell. It will help you practice more to be at the moment.

Walking

It is a daily activity that has brought more value to, by paying attention to it. You are to focus on the movement of your feet touching and leaving the ground.

Mindful Breathing

As breath goes in and out, you are told to practice to focus on the physical sensations you feel.

Build Compassion through Mindfulness

This kind of meditation is focused on compassion towards others and more importantly to yourself. The first step is to practice it towards you then slowly to your closed ones. It goes off like that then finally to people you don't really care about or have a negative feeling about them.

Mindfulness and Anxiety

Life happens to you as it does to everybody. It is not always the case of liking life but we always like to make it responsible whenever something bad happens. We should be open to experiencing good and bad aspects of life by taking them as they are.

Anxiety is part of being human. So many people experience it on the regular. It has not been recognized as a disorder.

Mindfulness-based therapies are solely about the relationship between the person experiencing anxiety and their thoughts. The relationship is not great, to say the least hence the anxiety, so mindfulness is there to try and change that.

A person is made aware and to confront the bodily sensations that come along whenever he or she is feeling anxiety. They are made to fully experience what goes on at that moment rather than trying to hide from it like they have been doing before. The withdrawing was obviously not working and it never does in case of anxiety. So it is better to buckle up and face the music. It is not only the physical symptoms they are made to face but also their thoughts. They are advised to open up to them. Experiencing all these thoughts will eventually make a person realize that they were not true, to begin with. They have been avoiding them for no reason and building up their anxiety about them.

The person practicing mindfulness will be taught to realize and respond to their distressing thoughts and then they will start letting them go. Not acknowledging them was the problem in the first place.

Breath-Control

Your breathing tends to become shallower as you panic more. So if you start experiencing panic then immediately start counting your breaths, while keeping your eyes closed. If your breathing has turned rapid then just focus on a couple of inhales and exhales. While counting, if your mind is not focused on breathing, then it means success. You have actually practiced mindfulness in a trying time.

Become Aware of your Body

When experiencing a panic attack, try to pay attention to your body and what is happening to every part of it. Try to feel your toes and fingers and sense if your muscles are tensing up. As you become aware of this feeling, try to let it happen and do not try to resist it. Just becoming aware will help you but resisting will make it worse.

Become Aware of your Surrounding

It is not always the case that keeping to your eyes while having a panic attack will help you resist it. More often than not, being aware of your surrounding helps more. So open your eyes and try to interact with your surroundings via your brain. Say hello to things present in your room. It will help you ground yourself.

By experiencing a nervous or stressing situation, an anxious person reacts to it which is usually via an unnecessary fight or flight response. It has no business in the majority of situations an anxious person is involved in. Thus by mindfulness instead of reacting, you are taught to respond to them positively. It is done by practicing to be present in your body and fully knowing what is going on that is giving you anxiety in the first place. You will eventually figure out it was all about a thing that you are perceiving and categorizing as threats. As you will find anxiety to be nothing more than a perceived threat, it will vanish on its own.

Mindfulness-based therapies are proved to be helpful in reducing depression. (Borchard, 2019)[7]

Some people find it impossible to just sit still for a while. Meditation involves staying still and could be a very daunting task for them. A worthwhile solution for them is to take a pause during the day and just take five deep breaths. That should do it for them. You can practice it whenever you feel.

---

[7] Borchard, T. (2019). 6 Steps for Beating Depression. Retrieved from https://psychcentral.com/blog/6-steps-for-beating-depression/

Sometimes it helps to practice mindfulness with a group of people. You will see you are not an outlier and everyone makes mistakes. That will help you stick to mindfulness and not to give up on it. Meditation is thought of as a solo activity, but more often than not it helps to do it while being part of a group.

Some people even have heightened anxiety when trying to sit still and meditate. It is advisable to let it pass and not let your determination waver. It is the key if you want to bring a positive change in your life.

The distressing thoughts that you are so afraid to face, once you let them pass without reacting, you will literally gain a new skillset. One that will next time guide you on how to deal with fear and anxious thoughts.

Mindfulness can make you see things more clearly. It will help you achieve inner peace.

Chapter 5: Meditation and its Effectiveness

"Someone asked Buddha what he gained from meditation and replied "Nothing. However, he said, let me tell you what I lost: Anger, Anxiety, Insecurity, and Depression, fear of old age and death."

Meditation for Anxiety

The mind is the most complex mechanism there is. So don't worry if you don't understand it. Meditation can help you get to know your mind better.

Meditation is like a new skill that you never used before and with just a little practice, you can easily hone it to make your life healthier. If you decide to take up meditation, then don't fret about results as soon as you close your eyes. You should bear in mind that it's the journey that matters and not the destination in this particular case.

Meditation isn't there to alter the person you are. It does not mean having an on and off switch for your thoughts, but rather a heightened sense of awareness. It allows us to develop a healthier outlook and be more positive in thoughts and actions. It can train you to expend no judgment and taking the moments just as they are.

Getting to know and basically acknowledging your anxiety is the first step you can take to handle it. Anyone who has had trouble with anxiety before can attest to the fact that it is a nerve-racking experience. You cannot simply make sense of it, let alone think of any ways to counter it at that moment. Now, this is where meditation will take the wheel and once you regularly and successfully incorporated it in your life, you will start to see real development for your mental health.

Meditation is a viable solution that is long lasting and side-effects free. Besides getting rid of anxiety for the lifetime, you gain numerous other benefits. All it requires is that you put your effort and dedication into it and not lose heart. Eventually, this practice will bear fruit. Meditation is known to have as much effect as anti-depressant medication. (Goyal et al., 2014)

When experiencing anxiety, we lose control of our emotions. Research has found that meditation can rewire the brain's neural pathways. This will help gain the upper hand on emotions and significantly reduce anxiety.

What meditation does is basically acquaint ourselves with thoughts that are causing anxiety in our brains. As we get to know them better, we realize they simply don't matter. Another thing to learn through meditation is that whatever our speculation is, and what really ends up happening, in reality, is not the same thing. The thoughts are all conjured in our brains due to insecurities. We learn what is real and truly matters. We then have a good idea about the irrational ruminations our brain has managed to come up with.

Meditation posture

1. You have to practice your posture for meditation:
2. Find a good place to sit on. You should not be perching on it or being uncomfortable in your seat.
3. Your feet should be stable. For example, if you are sitting on the ground, then your legs should be crossed. If you have chosen a chair to sit on, then both feet should be on the ground.
4. Your frame should not ramrod straight as it is thought of as a typical posture for meditation. Your spine has a natural curve and you should be sitting according to it.

5. If your upper arms are too far back from your upper body, then it will make you sit stiffly. And if they are too forward, you will be hunching down. It is therefore recommended to sit with your upper arms parallel to your upper body.
6. It is not important to close your eyes, but if you have trouble focusing while keeping your eyes open, then it is necessary. Other than that, you can also gently let your gaze fall lower by tilting your head a little downward.
7. When you are set and ready for meditation, start with following your breath and pay attention to it. After a while of focusing, your mind will be bringing your attention to other things and when you become aware of it happening, begin to follow your breath again. Don't worry about not being able to keep focus; it is a gradual learning process.
8. Relax for a few moments. When you get up to carry on about your day, you should feel satisfied with your meditation. It should feel a little different than when you sat down to meditate. If you feel the same or even worse, then you still need more practice to make meditation work for you.

It is one of those things that seems pretty simple but is not easy at all. The results will only appear after you don't give up on it, even if you feel like not making any progress at all.

Types of Meditation

There are different types of meditations that you can try and find whatever suits you best. Meditation can offer a long term solution to anxiety. You can even include more than one type in your routine.

Breath awareness

As the name indicates, it is a type of meditation that focusses particularly on breathing. It basically is a practice on mindful breathing. It is a mindful meditation type, so its benefits include a reduction in anxiety and better control of emotions.

You are taught to breathe slowly and deeply. Your sole focus is on breathing or counting them. By doing so, you are consciously ignoring all other thoughts that enter your brain. This is also one of the techniques to benefit from during a panic attack.

Progressive Relaxation

In this form of meditation, you are to do a scan on your whole body to find parts that are most tense, then coincide your attention and focus into that spot. It is to release tension from that place. This form of meditation usually begins from the toe and then worked our way up.

There are a couple of ways to approach it.

- Tense up and then relax your muscles.
- Another way is to visualize a wave and imagine it passing over your body. When it does so, tension in your body also dissipates.

This meditation is for achieving a sense of peace not only for the mind but also for the body. It can also help people deal with chronic pain.

Loving and Kindness Meditation

This type of meditation is ideal for developing a more forgiving and generous attitude towards the environment. Especially, towards the people.

The first step is to open up yourself to receive kindness. Then it is extended from you to others. The key is to repeat the message many times until you feel like developing an altruist attitude. You have to be open minded for it to work truly.

Most people suffering from mental health disorders tend to have a less amiable attitude more towards themselves than others. Some find it difficult to let go of things. This is very harmful to a person's mental wellbeing.

Since this meditation promotes positive sentiments, it is good for general depression and anxiety. It can also help with post-traumatic stress disorder. Those who are affected by anger, resentment and unresolved personal conflict can truly gain from practicing this meditation.

Kundalini Yoga

It is a form of yoga where mantras and deep breathing are combined. Yoga is a proven activity to improve not only one's physical health but also their mental health. It puts your mind at a state of ease. It can also help with chronic pains.

It is recommended to join a class for it, but if you prefer you can also learn it from home.

Transcendental Meditation

It is a form of meditation where you remain seated and breathe slowly. What you are trying to achieve in your mind is to rise above your current state of being. It sounds like practicing for a superpower.

This meditation heightens a sense of spirituality and increases mindfulness. The practitioner is told to focus on a series of words or a mantra. Sometimes you can choose your own mantra. It can be something that you are trying to overcome. So by repeating it, your brain opens up to the said idea. In the future, you will be better equipped mentally to face that particular task.

Zen Meditation

It is a form of Buddhist practice also known as zazen. It is a sort of meditation that could be best learned by a teacher because of its various steps, etc. It is a more disciplined version of mindfulness meditation. If you want to delve deeper into your spiritual side besides relaxation, then this type is recommended.

What you need to do is to sit comfortably, close your eyes and really observe your thoughts. Let them play out in your head without passing any evaluation or judgments.

Meditation and panic attack

A panic attack includes 'attack' in its name for a reason. It is mostly because you feel like attacked as if you are in a horror movie inside your brain. Your body experiences all of the signs of fear. It can convert your healthy lifestyle to mere survival. Fear is encoded in a small part of the brain called amygdala. That is where emotions are dealt with. With constant anxiety and fear, amygdala becomes hypersensitive and hyperactive.

With meditation, we also get to be more aware of our bodies. We learn the all-important body awareness skill. It can be acquired by paying attention to all parts of your body. Same as we got to know our thoughts, we will learn to know our body's sensations by harmonizing with our body. We will learn to control a panic attack better and mitigate anxiety.

What meditation can do for panic attacks is to decrease the activeness of the amygdala, making it less frantic than before. Meditation can help us reset some amok parts of the brain so that we can regulate our feelings and thoughts better. This way we can successfully counteract panic attacks.

How to meditate to relieve anxiety

Anxiety and meditation are linked to the brain. Anxiety leads to a change in structure and chemicals in the brain. Meditation also does that but in a healthier way. Meditation has been proven to help a person relax for hundreds of years. A study was conducted to find out the uses of mindfulness meditation. Its number one use was listed as anxiety relief. (Goyal et al., 2014)[8]

There are several types of meditation for stress and anxiety relief.

- Unstructured and structured meditation:

[8] Goyal, M., Singh, S., Sibinga, E., Gould, N., Rowland-Seymour, A., & Sharma, R. et al. (2014). Meditation Programs for Psychological Stress and Well-being: A Systematic Review and Meta-analysis. Deutsche Zeitschrift Für Akupunktur, 57(3), 26-27. doi: 10.1016/j.dza.2014.07.007

In structured meditation, you try to maintain all your focus on a single object. It is something that you hold on to as an anchor for your thoughts. So when they wander and you become aware of them roaming, you can redirect to the object.

In unstructured meditation, you don't try to focus on anything. You face all the thoughts and emotions as they happen to you. You don't latch on to anything though and let them pass.

- Mindset meditation:

Visualizations are used in this type of meditation. It is where you create an image in your brain, of a life consisting of your values and aspirations. Once you start concentrating on your goals and values, your brain starts putting anxiety behind you.

- **Breathing meditations**

It is where you focus on your breathing. You have to practice breathing slowly and deeply. Breathing this way is also healthy for your body. You have to count your breath for concentration in this meditation. You can breathe silently or out loud. It will help you deal with panic attacks and anxiety.

- **Mantra Meditation:**

As explained above, it uses an affirmative phrase or word. They will help you reshape your thoughts. It also helps you think clearly, which anxiety doesn't let you do.

Benefits of meditation

1. It can obstruct the obsessive and nervous thought patterns that we have developed. Those who are familiar with anxiety know what a vicious cycle it is. It almost becomes a habit of a person. It is very difficult to break a habit. A habit, due to repetition, has stronger neural pathways wired into the brain. Meditation changes the way we respond to stress.

This is why you need to seek meditation in this case and put your trust in it. This situation is a forte of meditation.

With meditation, you will become aware of your thoughts. You will stop lapsing into the past and overthinking about everything with constant practice. You will learn new ways on how to deal with prying thoughts and eventually break free from the cycle of worry and stress. You are making your brain learn new ways to perceive and respond to thoughts. It will ultimately lead to being less panicky.

2. It will help us balance out our brain chemicals. The imbalance is what leads to the development of any mental health disorder. It is one of the causes considered for triggering anxiety.

Meditation practices can restore chemical balance. It helps with stabilizing the number of neurotransmitters in the brain. If you have a feeling of nervousness and on edge, it usually is related to having low levels of GABA.

GABA (gamma-aminobutyric acid) is a neurotransmitter that is responsible for helping us relax. Meditation can help boost its levels. It also elevates the level of serotonin and reduces cortisol levels. The former is required for feeling happy and the latter is a stress hormone.

It reduces chronic brain inflammation. Brain inflammation is related to increased cytokines levels. Cytokines are messengers and they modulate the immune response. Their elevated levels are related to anxiety and stress.

1. Meditation will help reduce inflammation. It can even alter the pro-inflammatory genes. After just eight hours of meditation, noticeable changes occur in genes that can be measured. ("Experienced Practitioners Reap Genetic Changes After a Day of Mindfulness Meditation," 2019)9

---

[9] Experienced Practitioners Reap Genetic Changes After a Day of Mindfulness Meditation. (2019). Retrieved from https://nccih.nih.gov/research/results/spotlight/111513

2. It can help us bring a healthier change in the brain. It helps with increasing the grey matter, especially the size of the cortex and hippocampus. The size of the amygdala is decreased. It becomes less reactive and that will help regulate anxiety. It enhances neuroplasticity and increases the flow of blood to the brain. As the neural connections between the brain increases, the healthier the brain gets.

Anxiety disorders are growing common as time passes by. The first step that people take to overcome it is to visit the mental health care advisor and seek medication or therapy. Anti-anxiety medications are effective for short term. No one wants pills to stick around for their whole life. They are addictive and can cause problems with long term use. Cognitive behavioral therapy is an effective solution, but it could be pretty expensive.

Chapter 6: Love yourself

"Your task is not to seek for Love, but merely to seek and find all the barriers within yourself that you have built against it." - Rumi

What is Self-Love?

Self-love means showing compassion to ourselves. You are not to be harsh with yourself and criticize every single thing. We often tend to do that when things don't go quite our way. Every time someone does a task better than us, we often blame ourselves for simply not being perfect.

A human being is made to make mistakes. But berating yourself on them relentlessly can cause serious damage to your self-esteem. The lower your self-esteem goes, the more likely you are to fall into depression and anxiety.

Practicing self-love techniques builds greater self-esteem. Better self-esteem is directly linked to good mental health. Self-compassion brings about these constructive habits.

Optimistic nature.

Lesser depression.

Lesser anxiety.

Putting the stress behind oneself.

We have to realize that mistakes and struggles are part of life. Those imperfections are what reality is. Self-love has some aspects to it, which are:

Humanity: To know you are just human and can make mistakes, but they don't define you.

Kindness: Like you treat the people around you with generosity. Self-kindness means also diverting some of that tenderness to yourself.

Mindfulness: Developing a healthy and non-judging point of view. It is about cultivating an open and curious mindset ("8 Powerful Steps to Self-Love", 2019)[10].

Self-love will give you hope and will help you pursue healthy behaviors in life.

Self-Compassion

Some simple steps for self-compassion are as below:

Recognize when you are giving into a negative state of mind. If anxiety starts to creep up, then it is time to call it out. Acknowledge that these feelings are affecting you. It's better to accept than shut it out completely.

Imagine if your loved one was going through the same thing, what would your reaction be. It won't be harsh and criticizing, will it? You will be kind and caring because you know they don't deserve it.

Rather than blaming yourself for your behavior, try to find an explanation for it and don't judge yourself immediately. Everything is not always black and white. It is our anxiety that tends to make us feel vulnerable and not be comfortable with ourselves and our thoughts. Making mistakes is common, but accepting them and promising to yourself to change for the better, is what real growth is as a person.

We often categorize ourselves to the lowest of the low and put others on the highest stage where they are practically flawless, which, in fact, is not true at all. Most successful people have owned to making great blunders. What they didn't do afterward is let those shortcomings of theirs to put a damper on their accomplishments. They believed in themselves and carried on.

---

[10] 8 Powerful Steps to Self-Love. (2019). Retrieved from https://www.psychologytoday.com/us/blog/the-mindful-self-express/201706/8-powerful-steps-self-love

If you have done something horrid, you feel responsible for, then it is not healthy to wallow in it forever. At some point, you have got to get up and think about what can be done to make amends. Those who love will support you, but ultimately it is up to you to make changes for the sake of yourself. You have to take the reins of your own life.

Self-love and Anxiety Disorders

Self-love is being patient and amiable towards yourself so that you can develop healthy habits essential for wellbeing. To find inner peace, it is necessary to practice loving yourself. When you truly love yourself, you can achieve true happiness. How can you be truly happy when on the inside you don't accept yourself?

Loving yourself is not to be translated into egoistic behavior. It is definitely not narcissism. Self-love doesn't mean you stop caring about values and do what you constantly want because that is what makes you happy. It is not built on the feeling of jealousy and envy. Those green monsters are opposite to self-care.

It is a feeling of being worthy of happiness. No matter what you do, you cannot escape your body. So it is better not to make it a prison for yourself. By being honest, accepting, and respectable towards yourself, you are truly allowing yourself to evolve into a better version.

If you don't love yourself how can you extend that feeling towards others?

Techniques of self-love for anxiety

Self-love helps in the portrayal of how you behave and defines your personality. Self-love promotes self-confidence. It can lead you to succeed at work and in your social life. It is one of the best weapons against anxiety. By regularly practicing self-love, you are sure to lead an anxiety free life. Self-love will readily prompt you to make healthier life changes. So by design, a healthy lifestyle keeps you away from anxiety and stress.

Most sensitive people are often prone to anxiety. Realizing that you are not what you feel is the first step to heal. If you feel overwhelmed, then this realization can give you a clear perspective and help you get rid of that feeling.

1. Get to know yourself better and don't be swayed easily by others' opinions of you. People who have self-love don't act in accordance to what others want. If you are in tune with your inner self, you will automatically experience less anxiety.

2. Surround yourself with people who truly care about your wellbeing. If you realize someone is detrimental for your mental health, then there is no shame in cutting away from that relationship. If you have a positive environment around you, it will help you more with your anxiety.

3. Practice conscious breathing. As soon as you feel like stress is going to get you and you will get a panic attack, talk positively to yourself. If you are facing a hectic schedule or any situation that makes you nervous, some positive self-talk is a great coping mechanism. Verbally outlay things you need to do and ensure yourself that you will get through it.

4. Indulge yourself in self-soothing habits, such as running a scented bath or using a calming scent in your house. Put on your favorite show. Get in the comfiest outfit that you can find. Seek warmth, sit by a cozy fireplace.

5. Enjoy some superfoods. They will impact your blood sugars and energy levels. It will help regulate those. Food impacts our brain and thus our mood also. Some of these superfoods are below.

- Almonds
- Chocolate
- Berries

6. There is a phenomenon known as 'Biophilia.' It explains that humans feel calmer and stress-free in nature. So try to connect with earth any way you can and you don't need to be a hiker or climber. You can tend

to a small garden or visit the park, etc. Playing with sand also reduces stress so just build a sand castle at the beach.

7. Acupressure has been practiced throughout centuries and people have documented its advantages. There are two acupuncture points located between the skull and neck. They are said to help with stress and anxiety. This is what you need to do if you want to try it.

- Place your thumbs at the top of the neck. It where the neck meets your skull
- Apply gentle pressure.
- The pressure must not be soft but firm. Keep pressing and throughout it slowly and deeply breathe three times.
- After that lazily float your hands in your lap.
- Then drop your chin to your chest slowly.
- In the end, take a deep breath and smile to top it off.

You have to start with love to get away from negativity. Anxiety triggers negative emotions like a shame for not being able to do things, not being able to handle situations and having a constant fear of anxiety attack. Anxiety is a one step forward two step backward kind of thing. You must have loads of patience. This is real life, not a movie where a single moment tends to make everything better. It is a good place to start your journey, but the real deal is the ride to reach that finish line.

How not loving yourself causes anxiety

When you don't care about your wellbeing, then it is called self-abandonment. It is directly related to anxiety.

Emotional self-abandonment is when you deliberately don't pay attention to how anxiety is making you suffer inside out. Loving yourself emotionally means you have a strong inner bond in place. When things upset you, rather than feeling helpless, you work it out with yourself. Anxiety will struggle to get hold of you if you start to practice true self-love.

Physical self-abandonment happens when we let ourselves go and don't think what is healthy for us. We don't sleep enough, don't drink water enough, or have an unhealthy diet. All of these things, if not resolved, are a one-way ticket to anxiety kingdom. Loving yourself physically means taking care of your diet and health. Health is true wealth after all.

Financial self-abandonment means that either you overspend and regret afterward or you don't spend money at all not even for your basic needs. When you do spend, you want to get the cheapest thing for fulfilling your need. You are not enjoying yourself this way and it can lead to unhappiness. Troubles with money related to debt are one of the biggest causes of stress.

Organized self-abandonment means that your schedule is a mess. You are not organized in your daily life. Being a bit mature and adult-like is helpful. Being organized and following a schedule are keys to success and will make you less prone to anxiety.

Relationship self-abandonment means that in a relationship, it is important that you resolve conflict not by giving in and going along with whatever the other person wants. You have to make them see what you want and then you both have to work on it. If you are constantly putting yourself down just to please others, it will end up doing you and your relationship more harm than good.

Spiritual self-abandonment is when you don't ask your higher power for guidance, wisdom, and love then it is likely that you will end up feeling lonely and depressed. Loving yourself spiritually means to stay in contact with higher power and seek peace within, so you can efficiently fight off anxiety.

Disadvantages of Low Self-Esteem

Low self-esteem is generally caused by not giving any regard to yourself. Having low self-esteem is often linked to anxiety disorders.

Social anxiety disorder

If you have low self-esteem, you are more likely to develop a social anxiety disorder later on. Low self-esteem can make one feel lonely. It highlights more negative aspects of your image to yourself.

Social anxiety disorder's main cause could be pinpointed as having low self-esteem. You built negativity around yourself based on some bad moment that happened. It affects nearly 7% of America's adult population ("What Are Anxiety Disorders?" 2019)[11].

General anxiety disorder

General anxiety disorder is often linked to having low self-esteem. It is a feeling of being unworthy. Self-esteem of a person develops by how they view themselves based on others' reactions towards them. People who are showered with lots of affections by others tend to have high self-esteem. Those who are getting rejected don't have a lot of self-confidence. People with anxiety disorder experience more rejection from their surroundings; some of it is all in their heads though. They will also be loved, but they fail to see it. 2% of the American adult population is affected by this mental health disorder ("What Are Anxiety Disorders?" 2019)[12].

You should evaluate how much people stand by you and how much they neglect you. One important question is how much do they matter to you? If they don't matter to you, then their rejection doesn't hold a lot of meaning. If they are closer ones, then it is usually stress and anxiety that is pushing them away. Seeking therapy for GAD will help you improve your relationships.

People with anxiety and low self-esteem become stuck and inactive. They feel demoralized to perform an action because of all the negative reasons they have

[11] What Are Anxiety Disorders?. (2019). Retrieved from https://www.psychiatry.org/patients-families/anxiety-disorders/what-are-anxiety-disorders

[12] What Are Anxiety Disorders? (2019). Retrieved from https://www.psychiatry.org/patients-families/anxiety-disorders/what-are-anxiety-disorders

conjured in their mind. General anxiety disorder will hinder your ability to take action.

Remember to acknowledge your accomplishments and thinking back to them will give you motivation.

Advantages of self-love

As you get more confident in ourselves, you tend to delay tasks, less in favor of perfection, as you did before. You develop a go-getter attitude that helps you pursue talks more easily.

We don't let failure get us down. We know setbacks are not intended to be mulled over, but to learn from and move on.

We learn to not let criticism get to us. We acknowledge negative feedback, but we don't take it as a personal attack. We get to approach it with an open mind.

Chapter 7 - Opening up about your Anxiety

"What mental health needs is more candor, more sunlight, and more unashamed conversation." - Glenn Close

Talking about it

Often something occupies the mind that causes you to worry and stress. If you feel helpless about it, it tends to put you under mental stress. Usually, talking about it and letting in someone else helps to ease the burden. It makes you feel less anxious about the problem. You usually talk to someone you trust. Their positive response and assurance uplift you significantly.

Suffering from anxiety is taxing on the mind and spirit of a person. A way to deal with it is talking about your stresses to people you feel comfortable with. A listening ear is sometimes all you need. If you feel like you cannot open up about it to someone close to you, then search up helplines especially for it.

Some people suffer for years with anxiety or any mental health issue and they fail to recognize it. Different people going through mental health issues have different experiences with it. Talking about anxiety and panic attacks also makes the person realize that they are not alone in this feeling. Loneliness breeds depression and it directly leads to anxiety.

The person you decide to open up to could be anyone, a loved one who supports you, a counselor, or an online professional. Those who have social anxiety will find this solution more difficult to carry out. The main reason why an anxious person feels like their relationships are suffering is that they don't have honest communication with the other person.

Those who share their experiences with anxiety online find it positive that people relate to them and there is no confusion about anxiety on their part. The main drawback you feel from talking about it to someone close is that they will never get how you truly feel. The only way to overcome it is to take a chance and trust them when they show open support towards you; you will feel a lot better than before.

Things to consider

Some people find talking about anxiety, a positive way to deal with it. People suffering from anxiety always have a negative inner monologue going on. So it's better to put a halt to it and channel that conversation with someone who is actually helpful.

There are of course some things to be mindful about while talking about this specific issue. Anxiety is not an easygoing conversation topic.

1. Evaluate your relationship with the person you are going to rely on. How they generally are will tell you whether they will support you or not. Otherwise, talking to them will do more harm than good.
2. Pick someone whom you have known for a long time. A close family member or a best friend will do. Picking someone who doesn't have a deep relationship with you is not a good option. It might even affect your relationship with them.
3. If you have decided to share your experiences with people around you, then consider the level of details you are going to give. If you are telling someone close then, it helps to give them more information so they can understand you. While if you are talking about it with your colleagues or general friends then just telling them some symptoms will do.
4. Think about what you are going to say. Talking about it will make you nervous, so being prepared in advance will help.
5. Don't think prematurely that they would be aware of the issue and instantly understand you. Some people who never faced it before will try to hold a discussion with you and ask questions. So be patient and answer them accordingly.

Accept their response but be patient with it. Don't jump the gun and presume that they have run off. If this is a new thing, then they need to adjust their emotions around you accordingly. Whatever their response is, just accept and move on. You decided to take the risk; it was going to go either way. If it works then kudos, if not then fair enough, you don't need to stick around them anyway.

Helping someone with anxiety and panic attack

If you have someone in your life that suffers from anxiety and you got this book to try and get an idea about it, then this is a special guideline for you.

1. If you see someone suffering and they want to leave the place, help them do so immediately. You can also remind them that they should put their health first and are not obliged to stay at that place.

2. Assurance is the most significant thing to provide someone during a panic episode. When someone is experiencing a panic attack, they often fail to think rationally. Telling them that it's safe and there is nothing to worry about is the way to deal with the situation. It is because the person having a panic attack finds it very hard to think things through and realize that there is nothing to be panicking about really. Assure them it will go away soon.

3. Someone who is panicking often forgets to breathe properly. It is important that you remind them to breathe properly. It is better if you help them through the process. Count the breaths and talk to them through the process. Tell them to breathe deeply and when to exhale and inhale.

4. Try distracting them from whatever it is that's causing anxiety. Try engaging them in a conversation about a topic that interests them.

5. Telling them to calm down or relax will make their anxiety worse.

6. Don't try to leave even if they suggest it. It's never a good feeling to be anxious and alone. Don't let their denial of gravity of the situation fool you. It is better if you stick around and see it through.
7. Don't ask them for an explanation but also don't treat the situation lightly. It's a traumatizing thing to go through. And if they have an anxiety disorder, don't figure that they are used to it.

Be calm, encouraging and positive.

When to see a Mental Health Professional

Anxiety is when stress response is triggered in a situation where it is not required. A little anxiety in often cases is helpful because a rush of adrenaline and increased concentration could be the difference in your success. Living with constant anxiety could feel like anything from distraction to outright being unable to function for the simplest tasks.

To gauge the level of your anxiety is difficult because anxiety is a normal emotion. It is not classified as a disorder on its own. Often when it worsens a lot to the point, it is apparent that it's causing serious mental and physical damage is when they decide to go seek help.

A functional impairment can present itself in a myriad of ways as a result of constant anxiety. Your world starts constricting around you. You will definitely become aware of it sooner or later. Here are some ways you can know it's time to seek professional help.

- If you are easily irritable now, then it is a big sign that anxiety has affected you a lot and changed your ways.
- If physical symptoms have started to appear.

You are deserving of having good health. If your anxiety is making you suffer, then you shouldn't play it down. Don't let anyone talk you out of it and definitely not overthink this issue.

Different professionals have their own methods. So if you are not comfortable, then it's best to change the doctor. A good therapist will help you gain trust and they will concentrate on you.

Here are some of the things you must keep in mind in order to evaluate your therapist.

- Listens to and values your opinions and thoughts.
- Help you learn the process of change.
- Wants the best for you.
- Challenges your negative thoughts.
- Encourage your positive thoughts.
- Evaluates your progress and asks if you are getting what you want out of your therapy.

Benefits of Talking about Mental Health

As time passes by, the stigma around the topic is dissipating. Lots of people are talking about it now and it helps to shine the light on a very important issue of the human psyche.

You must be aware that your approach to an issue is purely subjective and this fact may lead to you misevaluating a situation. It may seem a lot in your mind, but in reality, it might not be that overwhelming. An objective point of view will help you realize that.

It's how the saying goes "load off my chest" after relying something emotionally heavy on someone else. Carrying on your day with a head full of tensions and pent up emotions can cause a great deal of stress in your body. The saying is true, confining to someone will reduce the physical strain on your body. Here are some of the key benefits:

- Encourage others to share.
- Raise awareness.
- Share experiences with others.

- Be yourself.

You gain a fresh perspective on your emotions. Even if the other doesn't get it and just lends a sympathetic listening ear, you will get clarification about things on your own. Often when you say things out loud, they seem a lot less scary.

Talking Therapy

Talking therapies allow you to talk to someone who is actually a trained professional in listening and helping you through negative emotions. Talking therapy is not only for people experiencing anxiety but anyone who is feeling stressed and can't work out their emotions. They feel like bottling them is doing them more harm than good and they have decided to pursue some help with them.

Talking treatments can also be called counseling, psychological treatments, and psychotherapies.

Talking about problems will help you recognize them more clearly. You will know why they are there in the first place. You will see them in a clearer perspective and it will help you understand them and find a better solution. Talking therapies will help you get a grip on what is going on and come to terms with it.

Talking is helpful because thinking over and over about it in your brain won't do you any good. Anxiety can affect our relationships. So talking honestly to the other person will help you strengthen the bond you share and you will genuinely be happy knowing that they care.

Some of the talking therapies are:

Cognitive behavior therapy.

Dialectic behavior therapy

Psychodynamic therapy.

Humanistic therapy.

Support and information.

In the end, it comes down to your determination. If you are truly dedicated, then therapy will definitely work.

Anxiety and How to Talk about It

One out of four people is at a risk of developing a mental health problem in our lives ("WHO | Mental disorders affect one in four people", 2019)[13]. If you are not the one who develops it, the chances are that someone close to you will. There is no easy solution to overcoming them.

Walk and Talk Therapy

Walking and talking alongside your therapist will give you a better real-world perspective that could not be gotten from sitting in an office. It also seems more fun than that and thus way less intimidating.

Sometimes, the usual therapy lessons and medications don't work. Exposure to sunlight is good for mental and physical health. Physical activity is linked to better mental health. Walking is a not a very laborious but nonetheless very beneficial physical activity.

Talking therapies can help you deal with a lot of emotional problems such as

- Abuse
- Death
- Rage/anger issues
- Substance abuse
- Life-threatening illness

Talking is not all there is to it. Just like every other type of therapy out there, talking works wonders for some people and doesn't help others that much. But it's one of the most effective methods. When you make your therapist

[13] WHO | Mental disorders affect one in four people. (2019). Retrieved from https://www.who.int/whr/2001/media_centre/press_release/en/

understand you, then there is a much better chance of treatment to have a positive outcome.

Chapter 8: Misunderstanding and Mistakes

"Nobody realizes that some people burn tremendous energy merely to be normal everyday"

Misconceptions about Anxiety and Panic Attacks

Anxiety is a term that actually covers a lot of disorders. All of these group of disorders are based around some sort of fear. Although a large number of people suffer from it in one form or another, there is not a general awareness of how to approach the issue. Some try to ignore it altogether, while others make up their own coping mechanism and try to treat themselves by what they found online

People who throw out the statement "just get over it" have no idea what they are talking about. It is the absolute worst advice one could give a person suffering from panic or anxiety attack.

Just because anxiety is not diagnosed like other illnesses of our body, it doesn't mean it's not a real condition. It is wrong to assume that with anxiety, a person will fail to accomplish anything. Trying to avoid tough situations won't make you better.

The old brown paper bag trick is not effective according to new studies. It is a myth that breathing into a paper bag will help the panic attack. In fact, carrying the paper bag around will cause anxiety and it can bring along a panic attack.

Waiting for anxiety to go away as you get older is a mistake that most people make.

Although it is believed that anxiety is related to genes in some way, it doesn't mean that if a parent has a habit of worrying that children would also acquire it.

Indulging into unhealthy coping mechanisms, like drinking and smoking will give you respite, is also a common mistake. It will make your condition worse.

Some parents try to force their children, who are displaying anxiety, into things. There is a difference in encouragement and forcing someone.

Anxiety is not the problem but part of the problem. There are mainly other mental health things related to it that need to be addressed as well.

Social support will help to get rid of anxiety. Support can actually help but ultimately you have to step up to fight your own battles.

There is no one standard way that tells us that a person has an anxiety disorder. Some people prefer going out while others shut themselves; they don't sound similar at all.

Misunderstandings people have about anxiety

1. *Only medications will resolve anxiety.* There are also therapies that go along with it to ensure long term success. There are also changes in lifestyle that will help you eventually control your anxiety.

2. *Therapy treatments are not there to discover the root cause and work on that particularly to reduce anxiety.* It will not work, although it is helpful to gain information on the cause. Therapies handle more daily routine anxiety symptoms.

3. *Stress is not always the cause of anxiety.* So completely shutting down from your daily routine and making it utterly carefree and relaxing won't do you any favors.

4. *Anxiety doesn't cause one to faint on the spot overwhelmed by intense feeling.*

5. *Some people believe that since everyone experiences anxiety, then an anxious person should do what others have done to avoid it.* It is not true that there

is always a reason for anxiety. Generalized anxiety disorder is where one can feel anxious without any reason.

6. *It is not as simple as telling someone to relax and a switch will go off in their brain that shuts down anxiety.* Anxiety feels like a hamster frantically running on a wheel inside a person's brain; they can't just order their brain to stop doing or feeling things. It doesn't work like that.

Mistakes about Anxiety

How can you make your Anxiety Worse?

Living a happy and successful life alongside your anxiety is possible. You need to struggle for it relentlessly with dedication. There are several coping mechanisms for anxiety. However, it doesn't mean that if one thing works for one person will necessarily work for another as well.

There are some things that you might think will help, but in actuality, they are actually harmful to anxiety.

1. Drinking coffee is a daily ritual of many people. It can perk one up in the morning by making them more alert. However, it tends to start up and boost over anxiety symptoms.

2. Too much time alone is never a good sign. It only pushes us right down the anxiety hole, from we try so desperately to escape from. If you really don't want contact with anyone then turn to a public place, where you can be interested in any healthy activity.

3. Don't avoid the places that trigger your anxiety. If you constantly avoid them, it won't help you get any better in dealing with your symptoms. If you try and enter those triggering situations, then it will only make you better in dealing with it and lessen your anxiety considerably.

4. If your anxiety keeps you up at night, then avoid looking at the clock. It will only end up making you feel more helpless about the situation.

5. If you are tired of anxiety and feeling on edge all the time, then numbing yourself seems like a tempting solution. But over time, it will do damage to your health. You are inviting a whole other problem upon yourself, which is an addiction.

6. After a stressful event or day, we tend to find solace in a tub of ice cream. The sugar rush we actually get from it will only increase your negative feeling of worry and sadness. ("Ice Cream Causes Anxiety Attacks", 2019)[14]

7. Even the people with the healthiest of mental stature feel helpless and depressed after sitting through a brief segment of news. All the loud music and flashes accompanying the negative images could lead to one becoming sensitive and numb. So if someone suffers from chronic anxiety, they are advised to stay away from the television.

8. Don't push away your negative thoughts. Try to work them out. Don't dismiss your anxiety and brush them away like nothing is wrong. You might feel out of place and ask "why me?" eventually you have to realize that it is a part of you and it will take an effort to work your way through.

9. Going outside can refresh one's mind. It is very conducive in case of anxiety as it centers one thought and brings a sense of peace to mind and body. However, brisk walking and stomping your way through will only worsen the anxiety you feel.

10. Spending time with your loved ones can help with your anxiety. But be careful with the choice of people you pick to hang out with. There is a difference between those who support you and those you tend to worsen your condition.

---

[14] Ice Cream Causes Anxiety Attacks. (2019). Retrieved from https://raypeatforum.com/community/threads/ice-cream-causes-anxiety-attacks.11909/

Anxiety Inviting Habits:

Often, unintentionally you can pander to activities that can inadvertently cause anxiety and stress to pile up on us. If you realize them quickly and try to get rid of those, it is a very good news for your anxiety. Bad habits are usually easier to get into than good habits. However, it takes a lot of diligence on your part.

Don't deliberately create a schedule that is too hectic and will overburden you for the rest of the day. Even if you feel very productive, it is not a good idea to have a jam-packed schedule. If you are prone to anxiety, then try to include little breaks in your day.

Don't be late. When you are running out of time, the sensations you feel make you more susceptible to having anxiety or a panic attack.

Never having any time for yourself is a very bad habit. You are always doing things that drain your energy away. You need to also invest in activities that recharge your energy. Allow yourself to take a breather and step back once in a while.

Taking shallow breaths is another habit that makes the body react in a way that makes it way more susceptible to anxiety.

Limit your accessibility and learn to say no to everything that others invite you to.

It is also a habit of people to constantly remind themselves of negative feeling and thoughts. They feel the urge to talk down to themselves negatively. It is a very destructive habit.

Not getting enough sleep is one of the worst habits for an anxious person to have. It will make your symptoms so much worse. If you don't get enough sleep, it can cause an imbalance in your hormone level (Vollert et al., 2011)[15].

---

[15] Vollert, C., Zagaar, M., Hovatta, I., Taneja, M., Vu, A., & Dao, A. et al. (2011). Exercise prevents sleep deprivation-associated anxiety-like behavior in rats: Potential role of oxidative stress mechanisms. Behavioural Brain Research, 224(2), 233-240. doi: 10.1016/j.bbr.2011.05.010

Too much time in front of a screen is not healthy. It is especially worse if you are on social media all the time. Spending time on social media gains us nothing in return and takes away our precious time. Especially stop the habit of taking your phone to bed and lie awake hours staring at it. It is as bad as it sounds.

Try to have a proper meal, which means to sit down comfortably and enjoy the food. If you develop a habit of eating on the go and rush through it, then it will be adding to your anxiety.

Anxiety Trick

Anxiety disorder is the fear one feels when apparently there is no reason to do so and they are not truly in danger. People get afraid and then try to protect themselves from that fear. When they do that, it spells disaster for them in case of anxiety. This is anxiety trick.

Unfortunately, it's a very common occurrence that sets people back to square one. It is one of the reasons behind chronic anxiety. If anyone is struggling with overcoming anxiety and ends up with no actual results, they are constantly getting fooled by an anxiety trick.

Down below are some of the anxiety tricks that present themselves in various types of anxiety disorders.

- In panic disorder, anxiety trick makes you believe that your life is in danger. You will go crazy.
- Instead of conscious breathing or any coping technique, you freeze and hold your breath just as if your life is in peril. You will give up and flee.
- In specific phobia, you start to believe that fear of an external object will consume you, body and soul.
- If you experience obsessive-compulsive disorder, then you believe that littlest of things can cause the biggest of catastrophe. Like if you think you have left the stove open, then it will instill in you the fear that your whole house will burn down.
- Anxiety trick for OCD will let people readily accept their compulsive and obsessive thoughts and act on them. They will not rest easy until

they do that thing just the way they want.

- For the generalized anxiety disorder, you start to believe that living in a constant state of worry will eventually make you mad.
- You try to stop intrusive thoughts that are causing anxiety and instead of accepting them. You don't let your thoughts pass you just block them.
- If you have social phobia, then you believe that you appear so nervous to other people that they will make fun of you, embarrass you, and eventually cast you outside the social circle.
- Anxiety trick in case of social phobia will lead you to avoid social gatherings. It shatters your confidence so that you begin to dislike yourself and tend to shy away even if you do go. It makes attending the event much more of an ordeal than it ought to be.

You pass each of this fear expecting it to come true any moment, but it never does. But now you are more worried when this episode of fear will strike again.

It's one's natural instinct to protect themselves, and that is where anxiety trick takes advantage of you.

You will feel like the harder you try; it only seems to get worse.

What is maintaining social anxiety? The answer is that the person has taken the protective measures he deemed necessary in his head. This led him to believe it must be due to those which eventually saved him. So he will only try harder next time because they feel like they had a narrow escape from the calamity. When in reality the catastrophe was never going to happen in the first place.

A person eventually realizes that whatever they are doing is not helping their case but worsening it.

So how to get a win from this sneaky trick, the answer is to expose yourself and spend time with your anxiety. As you spend more time in its company, you will eventually start letting go of fear. After sifting through all emotions and thoughts, they will subside on their own.

The panic trick works in the same way. You get tricked into thinking that you are facing real danger.

- You tense up.
- You try to flee.
- You hold your breath.
- You resist it.

These are all the things opposite of what would be helpful during a panic attack. Your panic has tricked you into doing them. You can train yourself to better fight off panic attacks. They are explained in detail in the next chapter.

Cognitive behavior methods of desensitization are where you practice with your symptoms. Your only chance is to lose the fear you have of these symptoms of anxiety. Only then they will go away. Don' try to be sneaky yourself and fight the anxiety. Let it be.

Chapter 9: Taking Action against Anxiety

"You can't stop the waves, but you can learn to surf"

Action Plan to follow for fighting Anxiety and Panic Attacks

There are countless people who suffer from anxiety every day. Some have brief periods when anxiety renders them incapable of carrying out a task and think rationally about the situation. In other times, anxiety can appear without warning while going through your routine. Two people who experience anxiety cannot relate exactly to each other.

Anxiety is often brought on by emotionally charged situations and stress-inducing circumstances. If you have gone through the process of acknowledging your anxiety and now you want to take charge of the situation, you must know that it is not an easy task. It is an uphill battle. Saying that with perseverance and determination, you can overcome anxiety and lead a happy and prosperous life.

There are medications and therapies that will help you set along to the path for recovery, but in the end, it is up to you to take the reins of your own recovery. It is up to you to find and adhere to practices that will bring about positivity and productivity in your life that anxiety tends to purge away from you regularly. So these are some of the things you can practice to mitigate anxiety from your life.

Whenever anxiety starts to loom, you will start to get negative thoughts. It will constantly remind you of your failures. So a good practice to break free from this and halt anxiety right in its tracks is to take a step back and acknowledge all the positive things that are around you. It is not all gloom and doom as your nervousness was making you believe. If you experience negativity in some certain situations because of your anxiety, then it helps to look at the possible positives of the situation.

Writing down can help you with your experiences with anxiety. Journaling your thoughts is a very positive coping mechanism. It not only helps you get it out of your system but when you are in a more peaceful state, you can reflect on the emotions and thoughts that stormed over you. You can logically deal with anxiety.

Organize and set up a routine for your life. It will help you avoid cluttering which brings about unnecessary stress and panic.

Practice the techniques that your therapist has suggested. Whatever they may be, meditation, breathing or spending time outdoors. Make room in your life for them.

Practice healthy eating and exercise.

Don't berate yourself on feeling anxiety; it is normal. There are some grounding techniques you can learn to avoid panic and anxiety. There are also breathing exercises you can turn to whenever you feel a panic attack approaching. Worrying about future events will not make them right.

Try and will yourself to have a healthier perspective in life. There is always light at the end of the tunnel.

Don't ignore or neglect your anxiety. Try to acknowledge and learn awareness about it.

Here are some simple tips to avoid anxious thoughts that bring on anxiety and panic attacks.

1. Your mind is not hardwired to deal with things in a certain way from a young age. We do feel like that because we often find ourselves reacting to things the same way our parents tend to do. You should know it is

not the case. You don't have to do things the way your parents do if it's causing harm. You can consciously change and be flexible about your approach to circumstances.

2. We tend to overthink about things and without even realizing it, we are reacting to it and making it very personal. This is a very negative habit. You have to learn which things should matter. You choose the things that affect you. For an anxious person, you have to develop awareness to deal with your thoughts objectively.
3. You have to learn to let go of things and not let every other comment that others say get to you. It can cause a lot of problems for your mental health.
4. Getting close to yourself is a sure way to beat of anxiety as it often stems from the insecurity you feel in the first place.
5. Observe yourself, your thoughts, and emotions. Bring yourself at peace with your thoughts. Take a moment to relish in the state of calmness. Remind yourself that this is what your true nature is. You are not your scattered thoughts and anxiety. You will eventually like this side of you and consciously make an effort to get on the track to your true nature.
6. It also helps to keep the present moment as a sort of anchor to elude anxiety and panic. Taking a step back and observing the situation really helps with the stress that threatens to upstage your peace of mind. Practice open-mindedness and accept situations to move on from them, rather than carrying their emotional baggage for the future.

Getting Rid of Anxiety

Here are some of the things that can help ward off anxiety daily.

- Exercise daily.
- Incorporate meditation in your daily life.
- Find reasons to laugh. It will help you in finding relief from stress.

("Stress relief from laughter? It's no joke", 2019)[16]

- Cleaning could take your mind off of worrying.
- Try to spend time in nature.
- Humans are social creatures. Try to spend times in the good company of your friends.
- Aromatherapy is an amazing way to lower your stress level.
- Uncertainty about your future often causes anxiety. It helps to pen down your goals and look forward to taking steps in order to realize them.
- Eat plenty of healthy stuff and drink an appropriate amount of water.
- There is nothing worse than, what not getting enough sleep could do for your mental health. Sleep deprivation hyper-activates the areas of the brain related to emotional processing and sets of neural activity that imitates anxiety. (Ph.D., 2019)
- Take supplements to regulate the amount of iron and vitamin B in your body. They are responsible for regulating serotonin in your body.
- Chamomile tea is a great stress diffuser.
- Instead of watching shows that put you on edge, try picking up light-hearted and funny shows that make you see the lighter side of life.
- Recently, coloring has been coming up as a great stress reliever and people say it makes their symptoms fade away.

When you feel a panic attack approaching, you can practice these two very useful ways to deal with it.

- Relax your muscles. Start from one end of your body and finish at other. You can tense up one group of muscle at a time for a few moments and then release it after some more seconds.
- Just try to acknowledge the symptoms that a panic attack brings about.

[16] Stress relief from laughter? It's no joke. (2019). Retrieved from https://www.mayoclinic.org/healthy-lifestyle/stress-management/in-depth/stress-relief/art-20044456

Don't try to fight them but tell yourself these are normal panic symptoms and are brought about because my mind is causing them. Just stay with your panic attacks instead of neglecting and being stubborn about accepting it.

How to Guide your Responses

You can teach yourself to guide your response from the feeling of panic.

Acknowledge the panicky feeling. You have to tell yourself that *yes I am afraid at this moment.* It doesn't mean that you accept that you are in danger. Just accept that you are feeling incoming fear. Accepting and not resisting is the first and foremost step you have to take in order to recover from panic attacks.

Stop listening to decisions that are upcoming as a result of panic. Don't follow them yet but wait them out. It is recommended to get a diary that you can fill out. There are also panic diaries available online which are essentially more like a questionnaire. If your panic attacks hit you during an activity which requires you to remain in your current state, then do so.

Here are some of the actions you can perform to fight off a panic attack.

1. Diaphragmatic breathing. Where instead of making your shoulders rise or fall, you push your belly in and out which increases the area of lungs at the bottom that remains compressed because of your diaphragm.

2. Have a silent talk with yourself about your surrounding and encouraging with some light-hearted talk.

3. Panic attacks are not a thing of the present. They come with what ifs about our future and past. So try to ground yourself at the moment.

4. Try to become aware of any tense area of your body and work to release the tension from there by actively thinking about relaxing it.

5. It's okay to relapse even after trying out all the above steps. It's actually common, so keep in mind not to become disappointed and just start again.

6. Panic attacks don't last forever and you have to realize it in order to constantly remind yourself during panic attacks that yes it is going to end.

Here are some of the things that will help you bring calmness, even if you don't suffer from chronic anxiety. These are some of the steps anyone can practice if they feel stressed out.

- Anxiety gets severe when we let our thoughts run wild without paying attention and working with them. So if you find something bugging you, then it's better to take your time and figure it out in your head from different perspectives and angles. Don't let your thoughts put you down. If something goes wrong, it is very detrimental to accuse yourself. You have to be honest with your thoughts. It is very easy to accept negative criticisms upon yourself when things aren't going your way.
- Taking care of your physical health is just as much important. Try relaxation techniques; they can do wonders for you.
- Clean out space you occupy often, like your room and office. Put up things that bring peace to you. Let the sunshine in your house and in your soul.

Final Words

This book provides you help from each angle it could. Main techniques that are used worldwide to combat anxiety like mindfulness, meditation are all discussed in full detail. After reading, this book, even if you don't have anxiety, you will be privy to so many bits of pieces of information that will make your life much more stress-free and significantly improve your perspective on life. It will help with your motivation also. Even after all the information available to you, it is up to you to carry the advice from the book. Anxiety is challenging and ruthless; it won't back down easily, so you have to practice patience and determination. You have to go after it relentlessly as well.

Bonus Material: Earning - An Introduction To Earning With The Double Your Income Sequence

SECTION 1: THE SECRET OF FORMING MONEY HABITS (AND HOW TO ENFORCE THEM)

You are a collection of your favorite habits.

And, you have a niche set of habits that contribute to the money you can earn and keep, during your average month. Understanding the science behind these habits will help you positively influence the energy you spend on making more money.

A habit is a practice that you have used so often, that it has become an internalized, autonomic blueprint – a kind of default program for how to execute a specific action.[17]

Habits become damaging when they stop being beneficial, and instead, become uncontrollable, unintentional and contrary to your personal goals. Most individuals carry with them the burden of many bad habits, which inadvertently keeps them from forging ahead and achieving their income goals.

According to Charles Duhigg, the reason why we struggle with habits is that they are as unique as we are. There is no quick-fix formula.

In order to effectively change your habits, you need enlightenment on a better process, and, on your stuck behavior. Then you can change your *cue-routine-reward* cycle.[18]

---

[17] Habit, Wikipedia, https://en.wikipedia.org/wiki/Habit

[18] Duhigg, Charles, How Habits Work, https://charlesduhigg.com/how-habits-work/

Cue: a trigger that puts your brain in automatic mode and chooses your habit

Routine: A physical, mental or emotional set of actions

Reward: What you gain from executing the habit

With fresh ideas and an understanding of how to break bad habit loops, you will adopt powerful new habits that will help you double your income every, single, month.

SECTION 2: HOW TO CREATE NEW MONEY HABITS

New habits are how you will double your income.

This means you need to:

#1: Identify and break bad habits, to free up room for fresh practices

#2: Identity and consciously adopt new habits, until they become automatic

This guide is not about the first step. If you want to learn how to break bad habits, I suggest reading Charles Duhigg's classic, "The Power of Habit."

What you do need to realize, is that a number of your existing habits need to change, to make room for the ones outlined in this guide. You must become consciously aware of your *cue-routine-reward cycle*, and interrupt it to stay on track.

You can do this effectively by replacing your existing rewards, with your new goal to double your income. To create a new habit, follow this simple process.

- Identify the bad habit that must be replaced
    - Waking up at 7 am to be at work at 8 am

- Identify the harm it's causing
    - Rushing and feeling harassed and irritated when you get to work

- Understand and replace the reward from your bad habit
    - Instead of instant gratification from sleeping late, your mood will be elevated, and your energy levels will be high at work

- Implement the new habit, motivated by a stronger overall reward
    - Practice waking up at 5 am, arriving at work at 7:30 and easing into your day, to stimulate the positive mindset required for success

According to modern studies, it takes roughly 66 days before a new behavior becomes automatic.[19]

---

[19] Lally, Phillippa, How are Habits Formed: Modelling Habit Formation in the Real World, https://onlinelibrary.wiley.com/doi/abs/10.1002/ejsp.674

SECTION 3: THE 14 HABITS THAT WILL DOUBLE YOUR INCOME

Here are the habits you need.

Habit 1: SLEEP (You're Not Doing It Right)

Bill Gates, the co-founder of Microsoft, sleeps for 7 hours every night and reads for 1 hour before bedtime.

With over a third of Americans not getting enough regular sleep, most people vastly underestimate the importance of quality shuteye in their lives.

Over or under-sleeping exposes you to increased risk for chronic conditions, mental distress, stroke and heart disease.[20] According to a 2018 Poll by The National Sleep Foundation, excellent sleepers feel more effective at getting things done the next day.[21]

The first habit you need to adopt is simple – get high quality, regular sleep.

Set a time every evening to go to sleep and stick to it. You should be in bed an hour before, your phone off and all screens far away from you. Read for an hour. Then, go to sleep for 7.

Wake up promptly, 7 hours later. Not a minute more.

Sticking to this new habit promises you stronger immunity, the improved concentration at work and greater emotional stability overall. Consistency will

---

[20] 1 in 3 Adults Don't Get Enough Sleep, https://www.cdc.gov/media/releases/2016/p0215-enough-sleep.html

[21] National Sleep Foundation's 2018 Sleep in America Poll Shows Americans Failing to Prioritize Sleep, https://sleepfoundation.org/media-center/press-release/2018-sleep-in-america-poll-shows

ensure that your circadian rhythms function well, and you never have trouble with restless sleep or with falling asleep.[22]

✓	Adopt this positive sleep habit

[22] Mahabir, Nicole, How and Why Waking Up at the Same Time Every Day Can Improve Your Health, https://www.cbc.ca/life/wellness/how-and-why-waking-up-at-the-same-time-everyday-can-improve-your-health-1.4357391

Habit 2: EXERCISE (It's Not Enough, or It's Too Much)

Ex-President Barack Obama works out for 45 minutes a day, six days a week. Thirty minutes or more of aerobic exercise is done daily by 76% of all successful people.[23]

Aerobic exercise is the one consistent habit that will give you the energy you need to succeed. You should run, walk, jog, bike or take a class at the gym. Cardio gets your blood pumping, which is ideal for your brain and boosts your intelligence.[24]

The second habit you need to adopt – find and practice an aerobic exercise, daily.

Now, you need to pick 45 minutes to an hour, every day to get your cardio in. It makes no difference whether you do this in the morning, or late in the evening – as long as it is done every single day.

Consistency is how you will reap these many benefits.

Try to pick something that fits into your life, schedule and likes. You don't have to spend money, you simply have to get active. This means finding an exercise you will enjoy. Some people like boxing classes, others prefer to take a walk around the neighborhood.

✓	Adopt this positive exercise habit

[23] Cohen Jennifer, Exercise is One Thing Most Successful People Do Everyday, https://www.entrepreneur.com/article/276760

[24] Regular Exercise Releases Brain Chemicals Key for Memory, Concentration, and Mental Sharpness, From the May 2013 Harvard Men's Health Watch, https://www.health.harvard.edu/press_releases/regular-exercise-releases-brain-chemicals-key-for-memory-concentration-and-mental-sharpness

Habit 3: SOCIAL ENERGY (Here's One to Protect)

Oprah Winfrey, talk-show host, and owner of Harpo Studios meditates for 20 minutes every morning, shortly after waking up.

Meditation makes you more in-tune with yourself, how you feel, and how the world around you feels. It's great for focus, increased energy, decreased stress and lifts brain fog.[25]

The people around you have an impact on your energy levels. Successful people surround themselves with positive, go-getters – while the average person is drained by one or more toxic, or negative people in their lives. Social energy must be protected.

The third habit is – to meditate daily on how to optimize your social energy.

According to a Cigna Study, loneliness is at epidemic levels in America.[26] But this is never a good reason to allow anyone a place in your life.

Take a look at your connections and consider if they add, or take energy away from you as you meditate for 20 minutes every morning.

Extroverted, or introverted, you need the right kind of connections in your daily life. If you have energy vampires in your sphere, you must get rid of them to be at your best.

✓	Adopt positive social meditation

[25] Sun, Carolyn, I Tried This Oprah Meditation Hack Every Day for Two Weeks. Here Are My 5 Takeaways, https://www.entrepreneur.com/article/310039

[26] New Cigna Study Reveals Loneliness at Epidemic Levels in America, https://www.prnewswire.com/news-releases/new-cigna-study-reveals-loneliness-at-epidemic-levels-in-america-300639747.html

Habit 4: SELF-INVESTMENT (Knowing and Doing)

Albert Einstein believed in constant self-investment through learning, research and application of that newfound knowledge.

The day you stop learning, is the day you stop growing. And personal growth is what takes you towards income acceleration and success. Einstein knew that constant reading was critical to learning, but so was the application of the knowledge learned while reading.

He famously said that too much reading renders the brain lazy. To grow in his field, Einstein continued to study formally until he was 26, then pursued self-study. He was not, as many believe, a naturally talented genius savant – he studied, read and practiced knowledge.[27]

The fourth habit is – invest in your field of knowledge through reading and practice.

If you want to excel like Einstein, shift from consuming entertainment to consuming knowledge. This is easily done by dedicating an hour or more to reading and applying your newly discovered knowledge. Practice what you learn, to see the real difference.[28]

Carve an hour of your day, in the morning or evening to read a book and then realize its lessons. This can be split into 30 minutes of reading, 30 minutes of creating.

✓	Learn and practice new knowledge

[27] Shead, Mark, Are You Reading Too Much?, http://www.productivity501.com/are-you-reading-too-much/8874/

[28] How Much Did Albert Einstein Study?, https://www.forbes.com/sites/quora/2017/12/28/how-much-did-albert-einstein-study/#1595adeb28bc

Habit 5: DELEGATION (Focus on The Big Picture)

Richard Branson, Founder of Virgin and hundreds of other companies, is famous for his practice of 'letting go, to grow.' He delegates to focus on the big picture.[29]

Delegation is a habit that most people fail to practice. Instead, they try to do everything themselves and end up burned out, exhausted and depleted.

When you actively practice delegation, you become a talented multitasker, able to orchestrate and design your own career. It is at this point your income will inflate.

The fifth habit is – to practice delegation often and keep your eyes on the big picture.

Your career, or income goals, maybe the big picture for now. Knowing where you want to end up gives you clarity of purpose, and will help you assign what is not important to those around you. This must be done in all aspects of your life that consume your time.

This habit will kick in when someone makes demands on your time. Ask yourself if it contributes to your big picture. If it does not, find a creative way of delegating it to another human being. Make this a habit, and soon you will be surrounded by competent people.[30]

✓	Adopt the habit of delegation

[29] Richard Branson: Why Delegation is Crucial for Success, https://www.virgin.com/entrepreneur/richard-branson-why-delegation-crucial-success
[30] Coleman, Alison, Delegate Like Branson: Hire People Who are More Talented Than You, https://www.forbes.com/sites/alisoncoleman/2015/01/25/delegate-like-branson-hire-people-who-are-more-talented-than-you/#4ce10d27cb3d

Habit 6: MENTORING (Learning and Teaching)

Marie Forleo is a life coach, philanthropist and entrepreneur, who believes in the power of mentoring and being mentored, to become hugely successful.[31]

In fact, she uses connections to grow her business at every level. With storytelling and the ability to build a community around her lifestyle brand, she was named Oprah's *"thought leader for the next generation."*

Your ability to surround yourself with the right people will be the single most useful habit you can adopt. Most people never actively practice the art of conscious mentoring.

The sixth habit is – to practice attracting network connections that will help you excel!

Who do you know that could teach you something important? Have you ever met someone who you wanted to learn from? Teaching and learning is fundamental to networking, and the basis for all positive relationships, in a corporate environment.[32]

Every day, you should consciously invest more energy in stimulating and improving mentor relationships that will help you grow and succeed as a person in your field. Be ruthlessly selective about your friends and who you spend the most time with.

Allow others to mentor you, and be mentored by you, in a working environment.

✓	Adopt the habit of mentoring and being mentored

[31] Brouwer, Allen, Lavery, Cathryn, Why Marie Forleo Says This One Marketing Trick Is So Important, https://www.entrepreneur.com/article/305586

[32] Forleo, Marie, Networking For Introverts W/Susan Cain, https://www.marieforleo.com/2013/11/susan-cain-introverts-networking/

Habit 7: YOUR 96 MINUTES (This is Your Most Valuable Time)

Stephen King is known for his work ethic and ability to produce six good pages of writing every day consistently. He does this by following the same productivity routine daily. [33]

You need to have the discipline and consistency required, to do something for your direct productivity benefit, for 96 minutes a day. Why 96 minutes?

Science says that everyone has 96 highly productive minutes every day, a time window when you have the most energy and are at your best. If you harness this power and use it for your ultimate goal of earning more money, it shifts from possible, to probable.[34]

The seventh habit is – Spend 96 minutes a day working on your main career goal.

Discover when your 96 minutes kicks in. It might be just after waking up. It might be late at night when everyone else is sleeping. Find your window and use it.

Spend those 96 minutes focused exclusively on your main career goal. If that is to get a promotion, this is when you will plan and execute a strategy. If it is to launch a website, this is when you will put in the work.

✓	Adopt the 96-minute habit

[33] Cotterill, Thomas, Stephen Kings Work Habits, https://thomascotterill.wordpress.com/2012/09/13/stephen-kings-work-habits/

[34] The Rule of 96 Minutes to Productivity, http://sapience.net/blog/the-rule-of-96-minutes-to-productivity/

Habit 8: INNOVATION (Get to The Core of Things)

Elon Musk, the founder of PayPal, SpaceX and Tesla, is a known innovator and practices the Richard Feynman technique mixed with first principles, to stay creative. [35]

The underlying concept of this technique is to not try and remember, but to understand – because when you do, you automatically remember. It's a way to entertain new ideas and be creative in a way that promotes productivity.

Knowledge to Elon, is about understanding the fundamental principles of a thing, to know the trunk and branches before diving headlong into the details, or the leaves of an idea.

The eighth habit is – when learning something new, to understand its core first.

Applying this to your career will make you a forward-thinking innovator. For example, if you are a psychologist, you would benefit from learning more about neuroscience, because it is at the core of your field. Competency is all about strong, unshakable fundamentals.[36]

Spend 30 minutes every day learning something that reinforces how you innovate in your chosen field. Soon you will be questioning, brainstorming and seeing patterns that may amount to improvements you can implement.

✓	Practice innovation for 30 mins a day

---

[35] The Feynman Technique: The Best Way to Learn Anything, https://fs.blog/2012/04/learn-anything-faster-with-the-feynman-technique/

[36] Stillman, Jessica, 3 Smart Strategies Genuises Like Albert Einstein and Elon Musk Use to Learn Anything Faster, http://www.businessinsider.com/3-strategies-geniuses-like-elon-musk-use-to-learn-anything-faster-2017-10?IR=T

Habit 9: THE WIN-WIN (Mutually Beneficial Relationships)

Stephen Covey, author of the smash hit "The 7 Habits of Highly Effective People" advocated the importance of win-win relationships.

According to Covey, most people approach life with a scarcity mindset, as opposed to an abundance mindset. Because of this, social interactions become unbalanced.[37]

There are several types of human interaction, win-lose, lose-lose, lose-win – but none are as powerful or effective as the win-win. When you practice win-win interactions, your engagements are mutually beneficial, and people will enjoy working with you.

The ninth habit is – to practice win-win human interactions in your daily life.

When you do, you will find that people flock to you, because they see the benefits of doing business with you. When everyone benefits, you can succeed together.

This habit will cue when someone asks you for something. This should be your trigger to think about how you can make the interaction a win-win scenario. Covey says, to take consideration and courage into account, and to be creative in your problem-solving.

As you create win-win results, your influence will grow in your field. Remember that there is enough success around for everyone, and you can create it for them!

✓	Practice win-win human interactions

[37] Hussain, Anum, 7 Habits of Highly Effective People [Book Summary], https://blog.hubspot.com/sales/habits-of-highly-effective-people-summary

Habit 10: SPEAK UP (Know and Communicate Your Value)

Tyra Banks, ex-supermodel, TV producer and personality, based her career success on the ability to speak up, negotiate and get what she desires most.

She made a habit of speaking clearly, frankly and openly about her value with the people around her. Too often, we get stuck in the habit of remaining passive, and silent about our worth. Promotions and opportunities will pass you by because you failed to speak up.

The tenth habit is – to speak up when necessary about your value as an employee.

Tyra explains, that it is a shift from an 'I need' to an 'I deserve' mindset. Instead of explaining to your employer why you need a raise, you should explain why you deserve one. This is easily done by focusing on your value – or how you positively contribute to the company.[38]

This is another habit that will cue when you identify opportunities or feel that you deserve a promotion at your job. In meetings, be open about your contributions to the success of projects or initiatives. Speak up about how you, as a person, make things better.

Getting into the habit of communicating your worth to people around you, positions you for rapid advancement. If you cannot see and communicate your value, the higher-ups will not see it either. Be persistent. Have a clear voice. And do not get lost in the crowd.

✓	Practice communicating personal value

[38] Atalla, Jen, Tyra Banks on How to Ask for a Raise, http://www.businessinsider.com/tyra-banks-how-to-ask-for-a-raise-2018-4?IR=T

Habit 11: PAY YOURSELF FIRST (This is Ground-breaking Advice)

George Clason was the author who wrote the classic 'The Richest Man in Babylon' and taught people to pay themselves first, in order to gain real wealth.[39]

Imagine if, since you had started working at age 21, you had put away 10% of every paycheck. This is what it means to pay yourself first. Money saved and kept earns compound interest and grows exponentially over long periods of time.

People that want to be wealthy use this strategy to move from employed earning to investing. Investing money is how you break out of your income bracket altogether.

The eleventh habit is – to put 10% of every paycheck aside to grow your wealth.

It might seem like very little at first, but 5 years of putting away just $100.00, frees up $6000.00 for investment. It gives you options to supplement your salary as you age.

To start the habit, every time you are paid – immediately take 10% of that total amount and put it in a separate account. You cannot touch this money. It is there simply to exist and earn you money from long-term growth.

The pay yourself first habit will help you clear away your debt, and get you investing at a young age. Get into this habit early, and you will benefit from time itself.

✓	Adopt the pay yourself first habit

[39] Canfield, Jack, The Key to Wealth: Pay Yourself First, http://jackcanfield.com/blog/the-key-to-wealth-pay-yourself-first/

Habit 12: SIDE HUSTLE (Spend Your Time for Returns)

Rob Kalin never meant Etsy.com to be such a smash success. Initially, it was simply his side hustle, born from a desire to make wood-encased computers. [40]

Rob Kalin is a furniture designer who started Etsy as a place to sell his wares. It was a side hustle, an increasingly common play among Millennials. Some 61% of Millennials work on their side hustles once a week or more.[41]

This is usually a job that earns them money beyond their 9-5, or a personal project with income potential that they are developing. What is your side hustle?

The twelfth habit is – work on your side hustle twice a week.

On Mondays and Thursdays, or Tuesdays and Fridays you should dedicate a couple of hours to your side hustle. This is a second business, born from your creative or analytical talents that may become a solid earner for you down the line.

Scheduling in time to develop your secondary projects is important for personal growth, and increasing your income. Many Millennials discover that once their side businesses reach a certain level, they can either sell them or commit fulltime to their passions.

✓	Adopt the side hustle habit

[40] Green, Penelope, Scratching an Itch, https://www.nytimes.com/2016/05/05/style/etsy-rob-kalin.html
[41] Sophy, Joshua, More Than 1 in 4 Millennials Work a Side Hustle, https://smallbiztrends.com/2017/07/millennial-side-hustle-statistics.html

Habit 13: SUNDAY REVIEW (3 Hours to Financial Freedom!)

Suze Orman, a personal finance expert and personality, is known for teaching people to pick just one thing about their finances to work on, at a time. [42]

She called it the 'one and done' method, and it simplifies the huge challenge of getting hold of your financial situation. Many people find their finances overwhelming, and so never take proactive steps towards understanding and controlling them.

The thirteenth habit is – to spend 3 hours every Sunday focusing on one financial problem.

You might need to save, or clear debt, or better understand your expenses and how to curb them. Whatever you need, you will tackle it during a designated time, every Sunday.

When you practice the habit of reviewing your finances regularly, to better understand and control them, you will change your life.

Make sure that you pick only one simple thing at a time so that you can properly digest and institute changes as necessary. Spend the time learning and streamlining for your ultimate benefit, as a responsible financial planner.

✓	Adopt the Sunday review habit

[42] Financial Resolutions for 2017? Just Do This One Thing, https://www.suzeorman.com/blog/financial-resolutions-for-2017-just-do-this-one-thing

Habit 14: MINIMALISM (Know How to Spend)

Steve Jobs, Founder of Apple, was a noted minimalist and wore the same black turtleneck every day for many, many years.

Popularized by Silicon Valley, minimalism reduces decision-fatigue, a common problem in today's overcrowded, ultra-informed society. With so much information and choice out there, it is no wonder you struggle to make good decisions for yourself.[43]

The theory goes that you can only make so many strong decisions in a day. The minimalist habit, allows you to dedicate those decisions to things that matter, like spending for value.

The fourteenth habit is – to spend with minimalism in mind.

Consumer culture is not for the truly rich. Instead, these individuals spend more money on a single item of quality, than repeated spending on numerous low-quality items.

Get into the habit of spending money on quality items, instead of cheaper items that will wear and degrade. This will free up your time as you make fewer wardrobe decisions. Instead of spending your creative energy there, you will spend it at work, where it matters most.

Less items of higher quality will simplify and improve your life.

✓	Adopt the spending for value habit

[43] Steve Jobs and Minimalism, http://www.applegazette.com/ipod/steve-jobs-and-minimalism/

SECTION 4: THE GOLDEN RULE OF SUCCESS SEQUENCING

Your habits determine your behavior, but one thing is more important.

Focus.

Your attention is a form of currency that will either enrich or impoverish your life. That is why they call it 'paying attention.' Focus is the literal gateway to learning, reasoning, decision-making, problem-solving and perception.[44]

That is why consistent focus on your habits is the golden rule of success.

None of the people you have read about in this guide could have succeeded without an all-encompassing focus on their daily habits. Every individual here keeps a rigorous, personalized schedule that optimizes these habits.

Success, like your daily habits, is incredibly personal. Only you can decide when you have achieved a high enough level of success. And your habits are the stepping stones!

If you want to double your income, nothing is keeping you from it, but your habits. When you remove the bad and replace it with these powerful income-generating habits, you will immediately experience rapid change that will reshape your life.

That is why your primary focus must be a habitual practice, according to a personalized schedule. Without it, expect to fall back into bad patterns of behavior.

---

[44] Dr Taylor, Jim, Focus is The Gateway to Business Success, https://www.huffingtonpost.com/dr-jim-taylor/focus-is-the-gateway-to-b_b_4206552.html

SECTION 5: THESE HABITS WILL MATTER MOST!

According to a study from Northwestern University, a domino effect happens when you adopt one lasting good habit.[45]

In other words, exercising every day will encourage positive eating habits. In turn, this may spread to you getting better quality sleep and performing better at work. Management of these small, seemingly insignificant habits starts with internalizing just one.

I want you to pick a habit from this list to act as your linchpin habit.

Then I want you to dedicate the next 66 days to internalizing that habit, and when you feel capable, adopt more from this list.

Even if you struggle to adopt more of these habits, I want you to commit to just the one. At no point over the next 66 days will you, at any point, stop practicing that habit.

The first couple in this list have the most impact. They directly affect your daily performance. This is how you will naturally double your income in the short term.

Consider the domino effect active in you right now. But it is focused on negative habits. Switch to replacing them with positive habits, and you will soar!

The habits that matter most are the ones you learn to keep. Make them part of who you are, and soon you will leap an income bracket.

---

[45] Clear, James, How to Create a Chain Reaction of Good Habits, https://jamesclear.com/domino-effect

SECTION 6: WILLPOWER OR WONTPOWER: YOU DECIDE

The number 1 barrier to change is a mysterious thing called 'willpower.'

Those who have it are strong. Those who lack willpower are weak.

That is what we are taught to believe in our modern society. Your ability to resist short-term temptations is chalked up to your measure of willpower.

But you are never told what it is, or how to get it. How is it meant to take over, when you have no idea how it works?

Now I am going to lift the veil.

Willpower is little more than self-control. It is the conscious act of choosing what is right, over what is easy. It is picking cognition, over emotion. It is discipline.[46]

Willpower is a *habit*.

Right now, you habitually give in to your desires. What you need to do is replace this with your long-term plan for success. Say no to instant gratification!

Practice consciously choosing to focus on what is most important, every day.

If you don't want to exercise, use your willpower. Emotions drive your thoughts. Replace them with conscious thoughts that are more beneficial. You must exercise, to feel good today, tomorrow, this week. You must exercise to earn more and be better.

Practice willpower as a habit, and soon it will take over.

---

[46] What You Need to Know About Willpower: The Psychological Science of Self-Control, http://www.apa.org/helpcenter/willpower.aspx

SECTION 7: REGAINING YOUR FAITH IN FREE WILL

'But I have so much to do.'

'I'll begin after my major project is over.'

'I'll just let this week pass, and I'll be ready.'

It is human nature to wait for the ideal time to change. You might have bought this guide with the intent to adopt these habits 'at some point.'

This is because you have lost faith in free will. Free will is your ability to choose between different courses of action, unimpeded. Now, life is all about impediments, but that does not mean you cannot choose to be better. You can.

We are all made up of a unique blend of strengths, weaknesses, circumstances and perceptions. Your free will must be exercised in accordance with your make-up, within your unique context, under your special circumstances.

The price of freedom is struggling.

The price of earning more is learning to be better.[47]

Then being better – every day!

If you cannot be better consistently, hope is lost.

In this way, free will gives you the opportunity to be whoever you want, as long as you are willing to go through the wringer to get there. It will be hard! If it were easy, everyone would be successful and living these rare lives.

My advice to be something is to practice.
Start and start *today*.

---

[47] Dr Schwartz, Seth, Do We Have Free Will, https://www.psychologytoday.com/us/blog/proceed-your-own-risk/201311/do-we-have-free-will

Check Out Our Other AMAZING Titles:

1. Self-Discipline: The Inner Edge of Success

A Student's Guide to Harnessing Self-Discipline for Success in College

Why are some people more successful than others? Why do some people become more settled, satisfied, live happier lives, and accomplish much more in college than the great majority? What is the real secret of success?

As a student, you all want to be successful one way or the other, in and out of college. Not only do you want the same things, you all know what to do to achieve them.

And they all intend to do those things, sometime. But before they get started, they decide that they need to take a sneak peek at their Instagram and Facebook wall.

They say that "soon they'll read that book."

Probably 80 percent of the student population lives on "soon" most of the time. They fantasize and think and dream about all the topics they are going to read "soon."

And who are the people they are surrounded with on soon island? Other people also on soon island! And what is the main attribute on Soon Island? Lack of discipline. They all sit around exhibiting lack of discipline which got them on the Soon Island in the first place.

They ask each other, "Why are you here?"

The truth is, they can always tell their reason for lack of discipline. Almost the same sentences: "I miss my friend; I had to go hang out with him." "The best movie of the season was premiered yesterday; we went to see it." "I have to reply to this message from my friend."

They have come down with the issue of indiscipline which is undoubtedly fatal to success. Their intentions are good, but as like we all know, "The road to hell is paved with good intentions."

For you to be successful in college, the rule is simple – Have self-discipline.

Don't be undisciplined. Stop getting into actions that encourage indiscipline. Do the right things at the right time.

The difference between success and failure comes down first to discipline. Is there anyone disciplined and unsuccessful? Look around and answer.

If you're honest, you'll admit that there are millions of people who have sweeter desires but have gone on to do wonderful things. You can do what these people have done despite having their desires, and also do well - if you try.

If you put as much self-discipline into achieving your goals as you do in giving in to your desires, you would actually surprise yourselves. But you have to first get off that Island of Indiscipline.

Want to read more? Purchase our book on ***Self-Discipline: The Inner Edge of Success*** *today!*

2. Cognitive Behavioral Therapy

How CBT Can Be Used to Rewire Your Brain, Stop Anxiety, and Overcome Depression

Cognitive stems from cognition, which encapsulates the idea of how we learn and the knowledge that we carry. The things you learn are part of your cognition, and what you do with that information is included in that category as well. Cognition includes a wide list of information that you might not fully realize.

Behavior is what we do. It is how we act. The things that you choose to say to other people are all about your behavior. How you react to what others have to say will exhibit your behavior as well. Your behavior is all about your mind interacting with your body and how that interacts with the people and other things that surround you.

Therapy is any form of help, usually from a trained professional, to help improve on whatever the therapy is specified for. You might get physical therapy to help regain strength in your knee after having a serious surgery. You can also get therapy to help overcome an alcohol or drug addiction.

Throughout this book, we're going to give you the basis you need to start understanding cognitive behavioral therapy. The three together—cognitive, behavioral, therapy—all make up CBT, which is a method that is going to directly help you overcome the mental illness that you are hoping to treat.

Therapy can be expensive, and even if you do have the means to go through with this process, you might struggle to find the right therapist. Sometimes, you might live in an area where there is only one therapist within a close distance, but you don't have a vibe with them that you find to be helpful. You might also find that you are desperate for help and that you want a therapist, but insurance coverage isn't always good for this.

By reading this book, you'll be able to find the tools you need to help with overcoming your most challenging thoughts. We are going to take you through the steps to identify the root issues and come up with specific methods to get you through.

*Want to read more? Purchase our book on **Cognitive Behavioral Therapy** today!*

3. Effective Guide On How to Sleep Well Everyday

The Easy Method For Better Sleep, Insomnia And Chronic Sleep Problems

"A well spent day brings happy sleep." — Leonardo da Vinci

Are you experiencing the worst restless feeling? Has your doctor diagnosed you with insomnia, restlessness, sleeplessness? When the whole world around you seems to be in peaceful deep slumber, you are the one who is restless. No matter what term is used to describe it, the fact is that it is you who is actually going through insomnia, and nothing could feel worse than that.

So you drag yourself from bed in the morning feeling as earth, with its entire lock stock and barrel, has decided to perch on your head for the day. Yet you go through the motions of the day, though you barely manage to make it through the hours. By the early night, you fall on to bed hoping this night will be different because you're dead tired and nothing will keep you from sleeping like a log. It's 2.00 a.m. now, dawn is breaking through and there you are, still wide awake and ready to scream to the world because no matter how tired you are or how hard you have tried, you simply can't get to sleep.

While there are proven facts and evidence of the devastating effects of sleeping less, the investigations are still on to establish the exact nature of effects resulting from too much sleep. Some researchers argue that people who sleep much longer than necessarily have a higher death rate. Physical and mental conditions such as depression or socioeconomic status can also lead to excessive sleep. There are other researchers who argue that the human body will naturally restrain it from sleeping more hours than really necessary. However, with research still underway for concrete evidence of the effects of over sleeping the best path you can choose is to adopt a sleeping pattern somewhere in the middle. According to the National Sleep Foundation, this middle range falls between seven and eight hours of sleep during the night. Despite these statistics, the best way to ensure you receive sufficient sleeping time is to let your own body act as your guide. You can always sleep a little extra if you feel exhausted or sleep a little less than usual if you feel you are oversleeping.

Dangers of Sleep deprivation.

Though sleep is something the average human being takes for granted, it is also one of the greatest mysteries in life. Just like we still don't have all the answers to the quantum field or gravity, researchers are still exploring the reasons behind the 'whats' and 'whys' of sleep. However, one fact unchallenged about sleep is that a proper sleep is paramount for maintaining good health. The general guideline regarding the optimal amount of sleep for an adult range from six to eight hours! If you carry on with too little or too much of this general guideline you are exposing yourself to the risk of adverse health effects.

Though sleep is something that comes naturally to many people, the problems of sleep deprivation have today become a pressing problem with more and more people succumbing to chronic sleeping disorders. Unfortunately, a great number of these people do not even realize that lack of sleep or sleep deprivation is at the root of their manifold problems in life. Scientific research also points out that lack of sleep on a continuous scale can lead to severe repercussions on your health.

If you have been experiencing impaired sleep patterns for a longer period, you also face the risk of:

- Severely impairing your immunity strength
- Promoting the risk of tumor growth, as it has been scientifically established that a tumor can grow at least two to three times faster among animals subjected to severe sleeping dysfunctions within a laboratory setting.
- Creating a pre-diabetic condition in the body. Insomnia creates hunger, making you want to eat even when you have already had a meal. This situation can lead to problems of obesity in turn.
- Critically impairing memory. How many times during the day have you found it difficult to remember even the most mundane and repetitive events when you have had no more

than 4 – 5 hours of sleep? Even a single night of impaired sleep plays havoc with our memory faculties, just think what it can do to your brain if you consistently lose sleep.

- Ruining your performance level both physically and mentally as your problem-solving abilities will not be working in peak order.
- Stomach ulcers
- Constipation, hemorrhoids
- Heart diseases
- Depression, lethargy and other mood disorders
- Daytime drowsiness
- Irritability
- Low energy
- Low mental clarity
- Reaction time slows down
- Lower productivity
- More accidents and mistakes
- Lower levels of growth hormone and testosterone

The growth hormone in the body which is vital for maintaining our looks, energy, and skin texture is produced by the pituitary gland. The specialty of this hormone production procedure is that it is only produced during the times of deep slumber or during intense workout sessions. In the absence of normal production of the growth hormone, our bodies will start on a premature aging process. According to research, people suffering from chronic insomnia are three times more susceptible to contract fatal diseases. When you lose sleep overnight, you cannot make up for it by sleeping more the next day. A night's lost sleep will be lost forever. More alarmingly if you continue to lose sleep regularly, they will create a cumulative negative effect that will disrupt your general health. All in all, sleeping deficiencies can effectively make your life miserable, as you already know.

How Much Sleep Do I Really Need?

This is a question that remains a mystery just like the questions of why and what makes us want to sleep. In response to a question of how many hours of sleep do we really need, an expert has answered that it is actually lot less than what we have been taught. On the other hand, though a good night's sleep is vital for good health, overdoing the sleeping can be equally bad for us. But if you sleep less and continue this for too long, the result will be confusion between body and brain signals, resulting in muddled thoughts, lethargic feelings, and overall lassitude. So, the question remains, how many hours of sleep do we really need? Is it essential to sleep the prescribed number of eight hours a day or is catching up a good sleep on a five to six-hour basis enough?

The eight hours of sleep theory is increasingly becoming unpractical in this fast-paced lifestyle. Actually, the recommendation of eight hours of sleep arises based on the idea that our ancestors had their beauty sleep between 8-9 hours in the past. In today's context, this concept is regarded more or less as a myth. In a study conducted by the Sleep Research Center, youngsters within the age group of 8 to 17 generally sleep for about nine hours during the night. However, in the case of adults, this theory is not applicable as a majority of them are sleepless and many of them thrive after a solid sleep varying between 5-7 hours.

A research conducted by the National Institute of Health has established that people who sleep soundly for nine hours a day or more are actually two times more vulnerable than those who sleep less in developing Parkinson's disease. A study report released by the Diabetes Care states that people claiming to sleep less than five hours or more than nine hours daily are the ones with the highest risk of attracting diabetes. In contrast, a large number of contemporary studies prove that people with sleeping patterns that do not exceed or fall beyond seven hours daily possess the highest survival rate. The persons who experience sleeping disorders and sleep less than 4.5 hours have the worst survival rate.

When ascertaining the correct number of hours you should sleep, the fact is that there is no magic number of hours. It will depend on a person to person basis as well as factors like age, activity, and performance level. For example, smaller children and teenagers require more sleep compared to adults. Your personal requirements will not be the same as your friend or colleague who is of the same age and gender as you. Because your sleep needs are unique and individual. According to the National Sleep Foundation, the difference of sleep requirements between two people of the same age, gender, and activity level is due to their basal sleep needs and sleep debt.

Your basal sleep need is the number of hours of sleep you typically need to engage in optimal performance levels. The sleep debt comprises of the accumulated number of hours of sleep you have lost as a result of poor sleeping habits, a recent sickness, social demands, environmental factors, etc. A healthy adult generally possesses a basal sleep need between seven and eight hours each night. If you have experienced sleeping difficulties and as a result accumulated a sleep debt you will find that your performance level is not up to its usual standard, even if you wake up after seven or eight hours of restful sleep. The symptoms will be most apparent during the times the circadian rhythm naturally alters like during mid-afternoon or overnight. One of the ways of easing out of an accumulated sleep debt situation is to get a few extra hours of sleep for a couple of nights until you regain your natural sleeping rhythm and vitality during the day.

Understand what Kind of a Sleeper Are You?

Sleep, dear reader, is the precious restorative that rights so many physical and mental wrongs. The elixir that transforms life and puts a spring in your step, a smile on your face, and the feeling that you can take care of everything that comes your way is sleep. Undervalued, ignored, and forgotten until you wake up to the realization that it's one of the essential foundations of daily wellbeing.

So what kind of a sleeper are you? There are many studies and descriptions of how we sleep but the common consensus settles for the following five simple categories:

1. Lively, healthy early risers!

These happy individuals usually get the sleep they need and rarely feel exhausted or fatigued. They are typically younger than the other groups, usually married or with a long-term partner, working full-time and definitely a morning person with no serious medical conditions.

2. Relaxed and retired seniors.

This is the oldest group in the survey with half of the sample being 65 or older. They sleep the most with an average of 7.3 hours per night compared to 6.8 across all groups. Sleep disorders are rare even though there is a significant proportion with at least one medical disorder.

3. Dozing drones.

These busy people are usually married/partnered and employed but they often work much longer than forty hours a week. Frequently working up to the hour when they go to bed, they get up early so they're always short of sleep and struggle to keep up with the daily pressures of life. Statistically, they'll feel tired or fatigued at least three days a week.

4. Galley slaves.

This group works the longest hours and often suffers from weight problems as well as an unhealthy reliance on caffeine to get through the day. Shift workers often fall into this group and there is also a marked tendency to be a night owl or evening person. They get the least amount of sleep and are more likely to take naps yet, surprisingly, this group often believes that, despite the state of their health, they are getting enough sleep.

5. Insomniacs.

Here is the largest proportion of night people and many of them quite rightly believe they have a sleep problem. About half of this group feel they get less sleep than they need and the same proportion admits to feeling tired, fatigued and lacking energy most of the time.

So, which of the five groups do you think you fit into?

If you're a happy member of Group One, your sleep should by definition be absolutely fine. Don't worry. We've got some really good ideas to share with you to keep you right on track and we'll even add some special extra features to your nightly rest routine to maximize the experience. If you're not in this group, our aim is to help you become a full-time member of the healthy, happy sleepers' association! Membership is for life.

Group Three represents too many tired, irritable, and generally inefficient individuals whose quality of life is impaired because they're too tired too often. Their work suffers because they rarely have sufficient rest to successfully assimilate the day's events. Their home life is degraded because work intrudes too often and they're just too tired to enjoy the pleasures and comfort of a life away from work. Feeling tired becomes their default position and they know they need to do something to give their minds and bodies the rest they deserve. Individuals in this group frequently suffer from long- term mental, physical and emotional stress.

The fourth group is rightly described as the night owls. They work the longest hours and, as we noted above, they typically work shifts. The health problems associated with this group include a marked tendency towards obesity as well as a range of inflammatory diseases. Despite the fact that these people rarely look or feel well, they seem to ignore the evidence and usually claim to get enough sleep, relying on sugary energy drinks and caffeine to keep them awake during waking hours. They take naps because their bodies can't function without additional sleep during the day. An objective analysis of their health would typically reveal a range of health and wellbeing issues.

Insomniacs are the dominant members of Group Five, people who don't get enough sleep, can't get to sleep, and who know they have a problem. Unfortunately, many insomniacs end up taking prescription medication to deal with their symptoms and we have to question the benefits of this solution in light of the many unpleasant side effects associated with long-term sleeping pill dependency. For insomniacs, life is a constant struggle because of the accumulative effects of long-term sleep deprivation.

Health issues abound, depression becomes a major risk, their ability to function normally is often impaired, and they lose sight of their potential to deal successfully with life's daily challenges. They sometimes refer to their condition as living in a nightmare world where they are constantly exhausted and simply cannot function. It's completely understandable that a doctor would prescribe sleeping drugs because the dangers of sleep deprivation can be acute.

Before we begin to examine the practicalities of sleep, we need to know how much sleep is appropriate for each of us as individuals. It's not surprising that different age groups have different sleep requirements.

For example, very young children and infants can sleep in total for around 14 - 15 hours a day. And if you've got teenagers, you might have guessed that adolescents usually need more sleep than adults. Teens can easily sleep between 8.5 to 9.5 hours a night.

It's widely understood that during the first trimester, pregnant women often find they need a lot more sleep than usual. The fact is that if you feel tired during the day, find yourself yawning or taking a nap, you're short on sleep. And this is the time for you to do something practical, realistic, and effective to take care of the problem.

There are many myths surrounding the condition known as OAS or Obstructive Sleep Apnea. It's estimated that around 18 million Americans suffer from the condition but the numbers could be much higher because many people don't report the condition to their doctors. This condition is far more than just loud snoring, although snoring can be a sign of sleep apnea.

People with this condition skip breathing 400 times during the night. The delay in breathing can last from ten to thirty seconds and is then followed by a loud snore as breathing suddenly resumes. The normal sleep cycle is interrupted and this can leave sufferers feeling tired and exhausted during the day. It is a serious condition, especially since it can lead to accidents at work, problems when driving, as well as increasing the risk of heart attacks and strokes. It can affect people of all ages, including children, but tends to affect people more after the age of forty.

Weight also plays a part and there is evidence that shedding excess pounds can improve the condition. Despite all the advice and overwhelming evidence, there are still surprising numbers of sleep apnea sufferers who continue to smoke. Smoking is a perfect way to increase the severity and risks of this debilitating condition.

If you've already trimmed your weight, quit smoking and tried sleeping on your side but still suffer from the condition, you need to see your doctor. There are many treatments available including a special mask that delivers constant air flow to keep the breathing passage open. Lifestyle choices can clearly make a positive difference, too.

Your body, your brain, your mind and your emotional functioning all rely on sufficient sleep to operate efficiently. If you don't get enough sleep, everything suffers. Research suggests that it's much harder than you might imagine to adapt having less sleep than your body needs. The sleep deficit has to be repaid at some point or we'll experience increasingly severe problems.

Simple techniques of preparing for bed

1. Try to get to bed early. The recharging of the body's adrenal system usually takes place between 11p.m. and 1a.m. in the morning. The gallbladder uses the same time to release the toxin build up in the body. If you happen to be awake when both these functions are taking place within your body, there is the possibility of the toxin backing up to the liver which can endanger your health very badly. Sleeping late are byproducts of modern living styles. However, the human body was created in synchronization of nature and its activities. That is why before the advent of electricity people used to go to bed just after sundown and wake up with sunrise.

2. Don't alter your bedtimes haphazardly. Try to stick to a pattern where you go to bed and wake up at the same time. This should be done even on weekends. The continuous pattern will help your body to fit into a rhythm.

3. Maintain a soothing bedtime routine. This can change from person to person. You can use deep breathing exercises, meditation, use of aromatherapy, a gentle relaxing massage given by your partner, or even going through a complete and relaxing skin care routine. The secret is to get into a rhythm which makes you comfortable, relaxed, and ready for bed. Repeating it every day will help in easing out the tensions of the day.

4. Refrain from taking any heavy fluids two hours before bed time. This habit will minimize the number of times you need to visit the bathroom in the middle of the night. You should also make a habit of going to the bathroom just before you get into bed, so that you will not get the urge during night time.

5. Eat a meal enriched with proteins several hours before your bed time. The protein will enhance the production of L-tryptophan which is essential for the production of serotonin and melatonin. Follow up your meal with some fruit to help the tryptophan to cross easily across the blood brain barrier.

6. Refrain from taking any snacks while in bed or just before bed and reduce the level of sugar and grains in your dinner time as it will raise the blood sugar level, delaying sleep. When the body starts metabolizing these elements and the blood sugar level start dropping you will find yourself suddenly awake and unable to go back to sleep.

7. A hot bath before bed is found to be very soothing. When the body temperature is stimulated to a raised level during late evening by the time you get into bed, it will be ready to drop, signaling slumber time to your brain.

8. Stop your work and put them away ideally one to two hours before bed. The interval between work and bedtime should be used for unwinding from the pressure and tension of work. It is essential that you approach your bed with a calm mind instead of being hyped up about some matter.
9. If you prefer reading, a novel with an uplifting story instead of a stimulating one like suspense or mystery is recommended. Or the suspense will keep you up half the night awake trying to visualize the end to the mystery!

A Few Lifestyle Suggestions to Make You Sleep Better

Don't take medications and drugs unless it is absolutely necessary for your health and wellbeing. A majority of prescribed and over the counter drugs can cause changes in your sleeping patterns.

Avoid drinks with alcohol or caffeine. Caffeine takes longer to metabolize in the body so that your body will experience its effects much longer after consumption. That is why even the cup of coffee you had in the evening will keep you awake during the night. Some of the medications and drugs in the market also contain caffeine which account for their capacity to generate sleeping irregularities. Though alcohol can make you feel drowsy the effect is very much short lived. Once the feeling goes away, you will find that sleep is eluding you for many hours and even the sleep that you finally reach will not take you to deep slumber after alcohol. In the absence of deep sleep, your body will not be able to perform its usual healing and regeneration process is vital for lasting healthiness.

Engage in regular exercise activities. If you are contained in an 8-hour office job, you should make sure that your body receives plenty of exercise which can dramatically increase your sleep health. The best time to exercise is, however, not closer to your bedtime but in the morning.

Keep away from sensitive food types that will keep you awake at night like sugar, pasteurized dairy foods, and grains. These foods can result in congestion, leading to gastric disorders.

The sleep apnea risk is enhanced amongst people with weight issues. If you think you have gained a few extra pounds and during this time you have also experienced sleeping trouble focus on losing the extra weight as a priority. The sleeping issue will correct automatically.

If your body is going through a hormone upheaval like during menopausal or premenopausal time, seek advice from your family physician, as this time can lead to sleeping difficulties.

Want to read more? Purchase our book on ***Effective Guide On How to Sleep Well Everyday*** *today!*

Bibliography:

1. DSM-5 Criteria for Diagnosing Panic Disorder. (2019). Retrieved from https://www.verywellmind.com/diagnosing-panic-disorder-2583930

2. Martin, E., J. Ressler, K., Binder, E., & B. Nemeroff, C. (2013). The Neurobiology of Anxiety Disorders: Brain Imaging, Genetics, and Psychoneuroendocrinology. Retrieved from https://www.ncbi.nlm.nih.gov/pmc/articles/PMC3684250/

3. C. Butler, A., E. Chapman, J., & M.Forman, E. (2006). The empirical status of cognitive-behavioral therapy: A review of meta-analyses [Ebook]. Science Direct.

4. Connolly, M. (2018). Anxiety and Caffeine - this stimulant in coffee or tea may fuel anxiety. Retrieved from https://www.psycom.net/anxiety-and-caffeine

5. Physical health and mental health. (2019). Retrieved from https://www.mentalhealth.org.uk/a-to-z/p/physical-health-and-mental-health

6. Smith, A., Chaplin, K., & Wadsworth, E. (2012). Chewing gum, occupational stress, work performance and wellbeing.

7. Borchard, T. (2019). 6 Steps for Beating Depression. Retrieved from https://psychcentral.com/blog/6-steps-for-beating-depression/

8. Goyal, M., Singh, S., Sibinga, E., Gould, N., Rowland-Seymour, A., & Sharma, R. et al. (2014). Meditation Programs for Psychological Stress and Well-being: A Systematic Review and Meta-analysis. Deutsche Zeitschrift Für Akupunktur, 57(3), 26-27. doi: 10.1016/j.dza.2014.07.007

9. Experienced Practitioners Reap Genetic Changes After a Day of Mindfulness Meditation. (2019). Retrieved from https://nccih.nih.gov/research/results/spotlight/111513

8 Powerful Steps to Self-Love. (2019). Retrieved from https://www.psychologytoday.com/us/blog/the-mindful-self-express/201706/8-powerful-steps-self-love

11. What Are Anxiety Disorders? (2019). Retrieved from https://www.psychiatry.org/patients-families/anxiety-disorders/what-are-anxiety-disorders

12. WHO | Mental disorders affect one in four people. (2019). Retrieved from https://www.who.int/whr/2001/media_centre/press_release/en/

13. Ice Cream Causes Anxiety Attacks. (2019). Retrieved from https://raypeatforum.com/community/threads/ice-cream-causes-anxiety-attacks.11909/

14. Vollert, C., Zagaar, M., Hovatta, I., Taneja, M., Vu, A., & Dao, A. et al. (2011). Exercise prevents sleep deprivation-associated anxiety-like behavior in rats: Potential role of oxidative stress mechanisms. Behavioural Brain Research, 224(2), 233-240. doi: 10.1016/j.bbr.2011.05.010

15. Stress relief from laughter? It's no joke. (2019). Retrieved from https://www.mayoclinic.org/healthy-lifestyle/stress-management/in-depth/stress-relief/art-20044456

Printed in June 2019
by Rotomail Italia S.p.A., Vignate (MI) - Italy